AF881594

GIRL'S ULTIMATE SEX GUIDE

THIS IS A CARLTON BOOK

Text and design © Carlton Books Ltd 2010

This edition published by Carlton Books
20 Mortimer Street
London W1T 3JW

10 9 8 7 6 5 4 3 2 1

Material in this book has previously appeared in *Satisfaction Guaranteed* (2003), *Complete Satisfaction* (2005) and *Man Management* (2003).

This book is sold subject to the condition that it shall not, by way of trade or otherwise, be lent, resold, hired out or otherwise circulated without the publisher's prior written consent in any form of cover or binding other than that in which it is published and without a similar condition including this condition being imposed upon the subsequent purchaser.

All rights reserved.
A CIP catalogue record is for this book is available from the British Library.

ISBN 978 1 84732 670 6

Printed in China

DISCLAIMER: Some of the text in this book covers risky behavior. Whenever precautions and first aid are mentioned and described in these articles, please be aware this is general advice only. This must not be interpreted as expert advice. It does not constitute a warranty that these instructions, if followed, will not result in injury. The information provided is of a general nature, and all erotic play is always exclusively the responsibility of the partners involved. Neither the author nor the publisher can accept responsibility for, nor are they liable for, any accident, personal injury, loss or damage (including any consequential loss) that results from using the ideas, information, instructions, procedures or advice offered in this book.

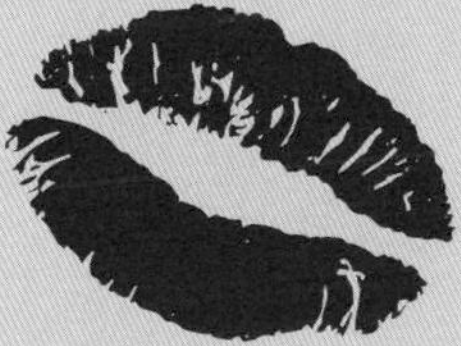

GIRL'S ULTIMATE SEX GUIDE

THE ESSENTIAL GUIDE TO DATING AND SEX FOR MODERN WOMEN

LISA SUSSMAN

CARLTON
BOOKS

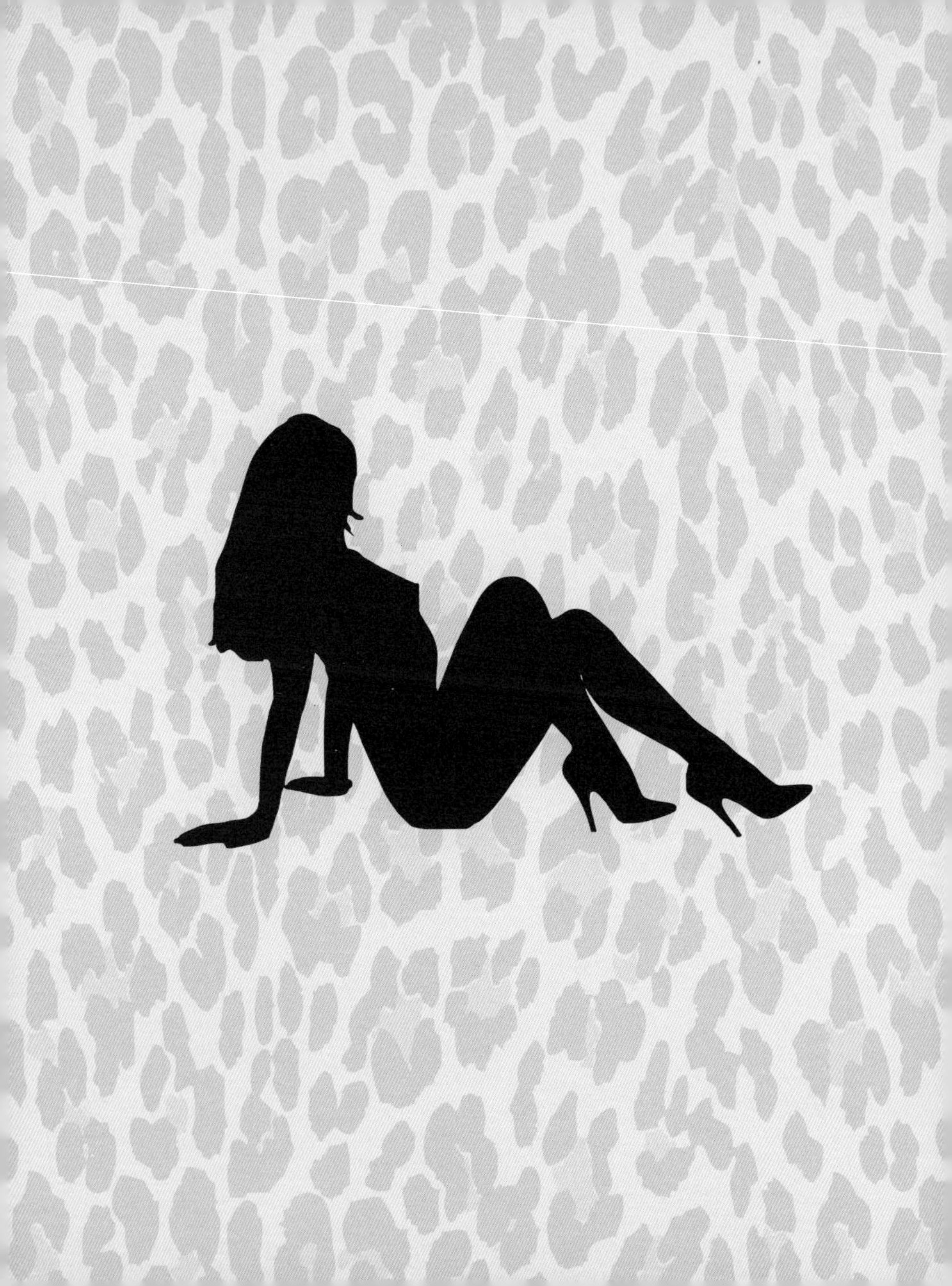

Contents

Chapter 1
Ways to Get a Man

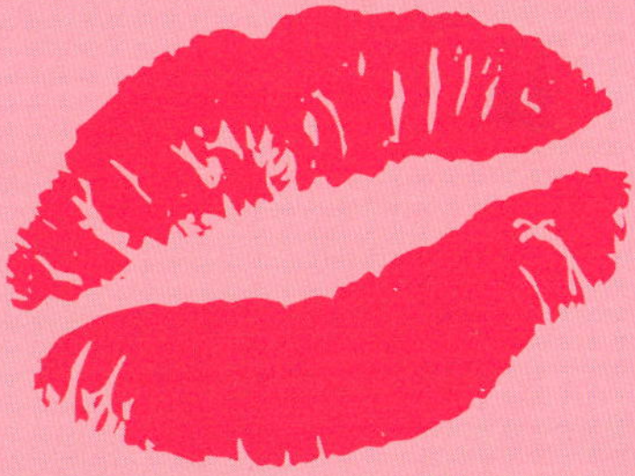

When You Only Have Three Seconds

Studies confirm that the impression you make in the first three seconds is the lasting one. We make up our minds in an instant about how sexy we find the other person. Here's what to do when you have just a few moments to grab his attention. Remember, though, while it's good to tune into your gut instincts, never put yourself in a vulnerable position with a stranger where you are on your own with him in a secluded place, and don't tell him your address.

Accessorize

Sometimes all it takes is the right prop to catch a guy's eye.

★ Use the novel approach. Certain books are guaranteed to put him in the mood to chat. *Fever Pitch*, *Zen and the Art of Motorcycle Maintenance* and *The Hitchhiker's Guide to the Galaxy* are all good guy-catchers.

★ Men are often more comfortable talking about – and to – big friendly dogs than they are about approaching a woman. So take your pooch – or borrow one – for a leisurely walk in the park. Bring along a toy and throw it in the direction of an attractive prospect. Or (accidentally-on-purpose) hit him on the head with your ball. That's sure to get him talking.

★ Grab your camera. When you see someone you want to talk to, hold up the camera and say, 'Fromage!'

★ Go fly a kite. And don't be upset if you can't get yours airborne. Keep trying until you spot the guy you want to help you.

Double Takes

Consider yourself warned: these five subtle, but totally sexifying, beauty moves will inexplicably draw every man in the area directly towards you.

1 Spellbind him with lips he'll lust for. A berry shade whispers seductively, while a deep vibrant red shouts, 'Look at me!'

2 Tempt him to touch you by massaging baby oil into your skin. Go out and enjoy your new high TQ (touchability quotient) by 'accidentally' brushing your bare arm against a cute guy's biceps. Instead of apologizing, simply smile – silky seductive skin means never having to say you're sorry.

3 Captivate him with your alluring cleavage. While a push-up bra can make your bosom perk up, a subtle golden shimmer will make it stand out among the masses. For a stare-if-you-dare divide, smooth on a sparkling sheer liquid bronzer from collarbone to cleavage, concentrating some colour in between your breasts to create the illusion of a deep, lusty neckline.

4 Eroticize your scent. If you want your scent to draw guys in like bees to honey, avoid the number one fragrance faux pas: perfume overload. Forgo heavy scents for a subtle citrus fragrance that he'll sneak up closer to sniff.

5 Tease him with lustrous locks. Catch his eye with the world's shiniest coif. Rinsing beaten egg whites into your head during your shower will add instant moisture, shine and bounce.

Give Yourself a Makeover

Knock-'em-out beauty is within your control.

★ Get a facial. Studies have revealed that the one thing that's guaranteed to make his head do a 360-degree turn is smooth, shiny skin (glossy hair doesn't hurt either). It's a sign of high oestrogen levels and difficult-to-mimic signs of youthfulness and fertility.

★ Dye your hair blonde. Research has found that blondes are more likely to be seen as eye candy than people with darker colouring.

★ Get dolled up. When a New Mexico State University study recorded beauty preferences, it was found that the look that made his eyes pop is a high forehead, full lips, a short jaw, a small chin and nose, big eyes and knife-sharp cheekbones. In short, Barbie lives.

★ Do your abs. A University of Texas study suggests that men prefer a 0.7 waist-to-hip ratio (i.e., the hips are roughly a third larger than the waist), possibly because it broadcasts a female's health and readiness to breed. For the record, Cindy Crawford and Naomi Campbell inch in with a 0.69 ratio. But so does anyone with a 70-cm (28-in) waist and 100-cm (40-in) hips – which just happens to be 47 per cent of the UK female population.

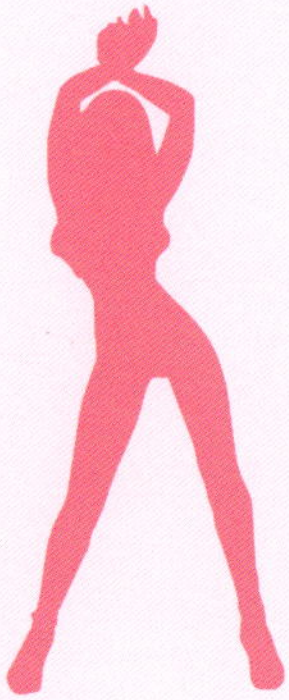

Scent Him Out

Smell is sexual chemistry in the most basic sense of the phrase. In a recent survey by the Fragrance Foundation, both men and women rated scent as an important aspect of sex appeal, giving odour an 8.4 rating on a scale of ten.

★ Follow your cycle. Researchers have established that a woman smells significantly different during ovulation – the time when she is most likely to become pregnant and therefore most needs to attract a mate – and that men are capable of sniffing out this change.

★ Use a green-apple scented lip gloss, then move in close. The scent has been found to work the limbic, or sex, part of the brain.

★ Stub out your cigarette. People who smoke are at a considerable disadvantage when it comes to smelling the subtle scents of sex. Smokers cover up their own natural scents, too, which puts others literally 'off the scent' – not to mention ash breath, yellow teeth and prematurely wrinkled skin. Bottom line: unless you're Bette Davis, lighting up cools his flame.

★ Douse yourself with lavender. Scientists have discovered that just a whiff of this fragrance can increase his penile blood-flow by 40 per cent, proving it to be quite the man-magnet. Other hot scent combos include black liquorice and doughnuts, and doughnuts and pumpkin pie.

★ Skip the perfume. Humans produce their own airborne, 'Here I am, come and get me' aromatic signals to the opposite sex. These are known as pheromones. Just stroll past and spritz him. Around the world, sweat is used as a love potion. An old Caribbean recipe reads: 'Prepare hamburger patty. Steep in your own sweat. Cook. Serve to the person desired.'

Follow Your Instincts

There's more to animal magnetism than meets the eye. Scientists have found that it's not that men are suckers for good looks; rather, they're genetically programmed to seek out a certain KIND of looks.

★ Stop dieting. Researchers at the University of Pennsylvania in Philadelphia showed pictures of female bodies ranging from almost skeletal to Rubenesque and found that it's not the men who plump for skinny women – it's the women. Biology dictates that women need a certain amount of body fat to produce hormones, periods and breasts (i.e. to produce offspring).

★ Go for an older guy – or lie about your age. According to a study of over 10,000 people in 37 countries, men are basically suckers for anyone younger than them (they equate youth with fertility).

★ According to the symmetry theory of physical attractiveness, callipers may be the only male-baiting accessory you need. It seems that humans, like most other species, show a strong preference for individuals who, when you draw a line down the centre of their body from their forehead to their toes, match up perfectly on the left and right sides. Studies have found that well-balanced babes have more – and better – sex than their lopsided counterparts. They're even more likely to have synchronized orgasms.

★ Look for your male twin. The reason why? Imprinting. People tend to be subconsciously attracted to replications of their parents. Hopefully they'll nurture you in the same way – only better. After years of trying to avoid becoming like Mum and Dad, we now look to date them.

★ Don't stand out. Studies show that from England to Australia and even in a sprinkling of hunting/gathering tribes, the facial ideal of attractiveness tends to be very middle-of-the-road. It's thought to be a prehistoric instinct that the more average a person is, the less likely they are to carry nasty health problems that will end up infecting the gene line.

★ Go pulling just before your period when your oestrogen levels surge. This is the Marilyn Monroe of hormones. It makes you feel finger-licking desirable and more likely to be chatted up.

Create Chemistry

You can't score if you're not playing the field. Ninety per cent of life is about showing up in the first place. Go out to places with signs of life – intelligent or otherwise – and use these tricks.

★ Dress like you're a success. When researchers showed photographs to a group of men of one particular woman, either dressed comfortably or wearing a business suit, the men rated the nicely dressed version to be much more appealing, without realizing it was the same woman. Talk about a power suit!

★ Make the first move. Ninety-five per cent of men polled said they would love to be approached by a woman.

★ A New England centre for the Study of the Family discovered that where you meet someone for the first time can strongly influence attraction. For instance, when men met a woman in the gym, they thought she was sexy and healthy-looking. But when they ran into the same woman at the pub, they rated her as unattractive.

★ Get in his line of vision so he notices you. Ninety-nine per cent of attracting a guy's attention is about getting him to see you in the first place.

★ Give up. That's right, forget about finding a date. Instead, start finding out what it is you love to do and what (besides the entire male species) fascinates and enthralls you most. When you stop waiting around for a guy to change your life, Mr Wonderful is most likely to show up. Ironic, huh?

When You Only Have Three Minutes

Your next move is the one that has the power to reduce a man to a trembling wreck. It's not beauty or even big breasts that attract men – it's knowing how to play the game. Make no mistake – flirting works. There's no better way to grab and hold a man's attention. Here are some sexy follow-up strategies for when you have a few more minutes on your side. Beware: these moves are guaranteed to turn even the biggest stud into a love-struck puppy.

Work Your Body

These body moves are sure to entice him.

★ Crossing your arms is a natural instinctive response when you're feeling vulnerable. The problem is, it signals DO NOT APPROACH. To avoid doing this, put one hand in your pocket, on your hip or on the arm of a chair. Or hold something like a drink or a pen (useful for exchanging phone numbers).

★ Working out is a great way to get male attention – not because you might meet guys at the gym (although you probably will), but because you will love the way a strong healthy body feels when you have the energy and ability to do anything. When you're comfortable with yourself, you inevitably come across as being more confident, sexy and fun.

★ Practise a sexy walk. Stand up straight, take a stride about one and a half times the length of your foot. This is the distance men are biologically fine-tuned to read as a sign of health and fertility, making you a hot prospect for passing on their genes.

★ When you slide onto a bar stool, sit with your legs crossed at the knee in what's called the Leg Twine. To wrap him around your little toe, languidly stroke your calf and let your shoe fall partly off.

★ Get the same effect from a distance by crossing your legs so they point towards a nearby cutie, showing that you'd like to enter his personal space (about 0.9 m/3 ft, according to studies).

No-Touch Seduction

Here's how to get a man to approach you without even lifting a finger.

★ Get a flushed face by thinking of something sexy or embarrassing. It's a signal to him that you're attracted to him.

★ Guys are suckers for long tresses. So entwine him in your locks by running your fingers through your hair and tossing it in his direction.

★ Scrub your tongue with a toothbrush every time you clean your teeth. Then let it slide out a little when your target is near. A healthy pink tongue is a visual turn-on for him.

★ Regular, moderate exercise alters metabolic rates and hormone levels, which often results in a greater sense of wellbeing and energy, an aura of confidence and an increased level of sexual desire – all powerful attractants.

★ When we first notice someone, we spend about three seconds scanning their face, flicking our eyes backwards and forwards between the other person's eyes, then moving down to the mouth and finishing off with a few broader sweeps. Extending the scan to four-and-a-half seconds will create strong emotions in him.

★ Buy time with a smile. Studies have found that when you smile at someone, they take a longer look because they are made to feel at ease.

How to Get a Man's Attention – Anywhere, Anytime

Now you've spotted him, here are some new, improved ways to catch his eye, start a conversation and keep it going.

ON THE STREET: Ask for directions – even if you live in the neighbourhood.

WHAT YOU SHOULD SAY: 'Excuse me,' which should then, in a millisecond, tell you how receptive he's going to be to you. If he seems to welcome the intrusion, ask for the whereabouts of a shop, restaurant or bar.

WHY THIS WILL WORK: Men love to be helpful (and act like know-it-alls).

POSSIBLE NEXT MOVE: After he gives you the instructions, say, 'I should write this down.' At that point, you should pull out a pen and paper and scribble down the directions. This will prolong the encounter, and if he's interested, he'll wait. If a prolonged conversation starts, since you already have your pen and paper out, you can ask for his number.

AT A SUPERMARKET: Ask him a practical question and allow him to help you out. Use the many hidden mysteries of the supermarket as a jumping-off point.

WHAT YOU SHOULD SAY: 'Do you know where they keep the crisps?' Then follow him around the aisles to find them. Or say, 'Can you reach that roll of paper towels?' or 'Can you believe how much this costs?' Or point out some snack choice in his cart (you'll have lots to choose from!) and say, 'Excuse me, but is that good? I'm supposed to bring something to a party later.'

WHY THIS WILL WORK: A direct question is always answerable and if he rebuffs you, you can always save face by asking the very next passer-by the same question (so your target ends up looking like a rude people-phobe).

POSSIBLE NEXT MOVE: More questions: 'I don't shop here that often. Is it always this crowded?' This leads to talk of his shopping schedule, which gives you information on his lifestyle (as does the contents of his cart), which can open the door to a million other topics of conversation.

IN A BAR: Stand near him, sip your drink and look deeply perturbed.

WHAT YOU SHOULD SAY: 'I might be going crazy, but does my drink taste soapy to you?' Hold out your glass to him. It doesn't matter if he takes you up on your offer to taste it. You've made the opening to say, 'I'm going to order another. Can I get you something?'

WHY THIS WILL WORK: It has nothing to do with talking about him, about you, or why you're both in the bar.

POSSIBLE NEXT MOVE: If he accepts your offer of a drink, comment on his beverage of choice. He wants a Bud? Say, 'Would you believe I tried draft for the first time recently,' which will launch a conversation about draft versus bottled. If he gets a cocktail, ask about the origin of its name, 'Who do you think Tom Collins was anyway?'

AT THE LAUNDRY: While fussing with a machine, surreptitiously drop a coin in such a way that it goes between the machines. Loudly express your frustration and attempt to pull the machines apart.

WHAT YOU SHOULD SAY: 'Oh no. I've lost so much money this way! I'll bet there's a fortune between these machines.'

WHY THIS WILL WORK: You've provided a conversation opener, and you've given him the opportunity to engage in a complaint-fest over the vagaries of doing your laundry. He might even figure out a way to help you get your money back.

POSSIBLE NEXT MOVE: Once you've been talking, ask him where he lives. (It must be nearby.) Then you can discuss the neighbourhood, the building and so on.

AT A PARTY: Look over and smile in a big, appreciative way. Smile as if there's a caption over your head that reads: 'I'm having a great time and I'm so glad to see you.'

WHAT YOU SHOULD SAY: After edging towards him over the course of 15 minutes, say, 'Hello.' Introduce yourself. Be a human being about it, it's a party, after all. You're supposed to go to them to meet people and mingle, so you shouldn't be too embarrassed to actually attempt to do so.

WHY THIS WILL WORK: Everyone's awkward at a party and he'll be thrilled to see a friendly, happy face.

POSSIBLE NEXT MOVE: After 'Hello,' traditional follow-ups are, 'What brings you here?' or 'What's going on?' If he has any social skills at all, conversation should ensue. Once you've been talking for a while (say, half an hour), you can always make the 'It's pretty noisy in here' or 'It looks as though people are leaving' observation and casually suggest moving on to another venue, like a place to get coffee.

AT A CLUB: Have fun on the dance floor AND look like you are, too. Often, when you dance, you're so caught up with what you look like or who's checking you out that you forget to relax and enjoy yourself. Then exit the floor, get a big glass of water and stand near the guy you're interested in.

WHAT YOU SHOULD SAY: 'I was wondering what the view was like from over here, and, please, tell me that I look pretentious/silly/ embarrassing on the dance floor!'

WHY THIS WILL WORK: A woman who doesn't take herself too seriously on a dance floor looks approachable.

POSSIBLE NEXT MOVE: He'll assure you that you dance divinely. Should mutual attraction happen, you could then say, 'Do you dance? Or do you come here just for the music?' If he wants to dance (and this is a huge deal for lots of men), he'll take the hint and ask you. If not, don't ask him, since his refusal could make for an awkward moment. And yes, we could ponder on why some guys go to clubs when they don't dance.

Oral Pleasures

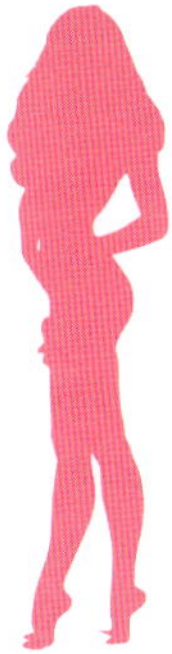

How to sweet-talk him with pick-up lines guaranteed to work.

A University of Louisiana study found that the following phrases will perk up his ears (and other organs):

- 'Hi.' (97 per cent success rate)
- 'Would you like another beer?' (91 per cent success rate)
- Introducing yourself (88 per cent success rate)
- Put your sweater or jacket down on the bar and say, 'Can you do me a massive favour and watch this for a second? I have to run to the ladies' room.' (85 per cent success rate)
- 'I feel a little embarrassed about this, but I'd like to meet you.' (82 per cent success rate)
- Touch his watch and ask, 'Do you have the time?' (81 per cent success rate)
- Instead of asking him what he does, ask him what he enjoys doing (78 per cent success rate)
- If you're at a party, walk up and say, 'Could I talk to you for a couple of minutes? There's someone I'm trying to avoid.' (76 per cent success rate)
- 'What do you think of the band/food/movie?' (70 per cent success rate)

Seduce him with your voice. When it comes to sweet talk, the pitch in which something is said is more important than what's actually being said. A softer, lower tone can literally stroke the listener, conveying vitality and sexiness even if all you're doing is chatting inanely about the weather. This is why, 'It's so hot' can sound finger-lickin' hot when breathed in a candy-floss whisper, and like a weather report when uttered in the monotone of a BBC2 DJ.

Tell him a secret. Disclosure gets him on your side. Lean in and tell him something personal – even if it's whether or not you're happy in your job. Men are attracted to that comfortable feeling of safety, so this makes it easier for him to share as well. But don't reveal too much about yourself.

When You Only Have 30 Minutes

Flirting is the most subtle form of man-I-pul(ation) there is. But playing hard to get is an art form that takes practice. Successful flirting is all about telling the truth about yourself but not giving the whole game away. Here are some man-baiting tactics for when you're pubbing or clubbing, or when you're at a party. And if you think they're too outrageous for you, remember: if there were no women out there who made the first move, most men would still be virgins.

Strut Your Stuff

Being aggressive with a stranger is a no-lose situation. If he's already noticed you, then he's thrilled; if he hasn't, then you're only making yourself less invisible to him. These no-holds-barred moves will make him look twice (and ask for your number).

★ It may seem polite to leave a little room between you and the guy you're interested in, but extreme flirting is no place for politeness! Lean in towards him to give him the impression that you want to exclude everyone else in the world.

★ Go for the kill by sidling up next to him and letting him feel your heat. Stand so close that you're almost touching him. When you step into his personal space, he interprets it as an immediate sexual invitation. If you stand close enough to a man for him to kiss you, he'll probably try.

★ Stroking your lower neck can cause your nipples to become firm. He'll happily take things from there.

★ Lick your lips when you look at him. Wet lips seem to simulate vaginal lubrication, signalling that he makes you horny.

★ Bump into him at the bar. Then, instead of saying, 'Excuse me,' put your hand on his back. Use gentle pressure, as if he were already your lover. When he looks to see who's behind him, say 'I'm sorry, I was just trying to get past.' Then flash him an innocent smile and move on. Guaranteed he'll be right on your trail.

Read HIS body moves:

♥ He chews faster
♥ His lips part slightly as he makes eye contact
♥ He touches his hair
♥ He touches his face more, stroking his cheeks, ears or neck
♥ He unconsciously (we hope) points at his genitals

Stare Him Down

Your eyes are 18 times more sensitive than your ears. Use them to captivate him.

The first rule men learn about picking up women is not to make an approach before they get the all-clear. One glance means a possible, 'Yes'. Two glances means, 'Come over'. Three glances and you're telling him, 'What's taking you so long?' Holding his gaze for two seconds is the magic number – any shorter than this and he can't be sure you're interested; any longer and he might call the cops!

★ Try the Two-Eyed Wink. A slower version of a normal blink, with all the playfulness (and none of the cheese factor) of a regular wink. Glance his way, then blink slowly and smile. Wait for him to smile in response, then look away again.

★ Try smiling with just your eyes.

★ If you're shy, gaze at his 'third eye' – the space between the eyebrows. He won't suspect a thing, but he will feel as though you are looking straight into his eyes.

★ Stay in the dark. Dilated pupils send out smouldering 'Notice me' messages, even if the distension is simply the result of bad lighting.

★ Short-sighted women have a peculiar attraction for many men, possibly because their unfocused gaze seems attentive. If you wear glasses, you can get the same effect by taking them off.

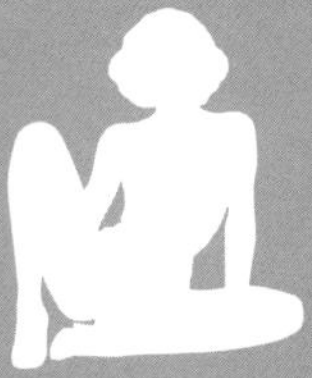

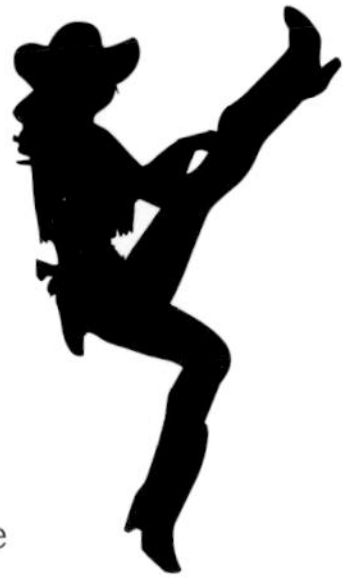

Be One of the Guys

Adopting certain guy-like behaviour will make him feel more comfortable about approaching you.

Know when the hunting season is. After scrutinizing birth records from around the world, German researchers concluded that there's a definite human mating season during the months when the sun shines for about 12 hours per day and the temperature hovers between 10 and 21°C (50 and 70°F). This means, biologically, you're more likely to look good to the opposite sex during these times of the year.

★ Hang out with just the guys: it makes other guys wonder why you're such a man magnet, and all that testosterone sends your flirty side soaring.

★ Drink beer out of a bottle. It tells him that you're down-to-earth and unpretentious, and he can be himself around you. (And that's not to mention the obviously erotic gesture of wrapping your lips around a long cylindrical object.) Cheers!

★ Ignore him. After giving him the once-over, pretend that watching paint dry would be more interesting than looking at him. It seems that while playing hard to get may be bad news for your reputation, it'll do wonders for your social calendar. Men are more often attracted to someone they have to 'chase' than someone who may be just as pretty, but more readily available. Apparently, having an urge frustrated can intensify the feeling of need, making him interpret it as must-have desire.

★ Don't leave until closing time. As the night wears on, magically, you become better-looking. In a study of singles-bar patrons, as closing time neared, people's judgement of a person's attractiveness increases. The reason: a psychological mechanism sensitive to shrinking opportunities. As the mating pool thins, what's left looks better and better. Of course, the next morning things may seem different!

When You Only Have Three Hours

You've attracted him enough to snag a first date. Now, make him yours. All a man really wants to know is that you like him. The trouble is, some women send out weaker signals than a cell phone submerged in water to let a man know they're interested. And if he thinks you're not into him, he'll want out of there. So, here's all you need to know to make him know that he is, without doubt, making your heart go flip-flop – without being TOO obvious about it.

Dress for Sexcess

Stylish moves that will guarantee he'll be ga-ga for good.

★ Wear something touch-worthy. A teasing hint of faux fur, a feathered bracelet or anything else that's tactile will catch his eye and make him want to stroke you.

★ Go *au naturel*. Using highly scented soaps and perfumes can interfere with his ability to detect your female scent, making him less likely to get turned on to you.

★ A poll by the University of California-Los Angeles found that guys regard a woman who accessorizes as a woman who cares about sex. The five top sexy adornments are: thumb and toe rings, charm bracelet, red cars, red lipstick and black stockings.

★ The colour of your clothes speaks volumes about you. In a study from Loyola University, Louisiana, both men and women rated red the most alluring shade, followed by dark blue, violet, black and yellow (virginal white didn't even get a look-in). Heart rates rise in the presence of strong red colours, so red actually makes him aroused.

★ Borrow his mum's clothes. The more you look like his mother or sister, the better your chances. It seems that after years of trying to avoid becoming like Mum and Dad, we now look to date them. A study from Rutgers University, New Jersey, found that people subconsciously tend to be attracted to replications of their parents or siblings in order to heal the emotional and psychological damage we all experience to some degree in childhood.

★ Call to him using a 'genital echo'. According to anything-that-moves watcher Desmond Morris, this alluring term covers all body parts with a passing resemblance to the genitals – in other words, a visual sexual double entendre. The belly button is one example, fingers another. (You figure out the matching genitals.) But the Big Mama of the pack is the mouth, which is thought to be a dead ringer for the vagina. In the same way as the inner labia of the vagina becomes bright red with engorged blood just prior to orgasm, our lips also become redder when we're turned on. Smearing your lips with red lipstick will send out an extra, 'I'm on the brink of ecstasy' announcement.

★ Wear a (figurative) mask. A little mystery is essential to infatuation. People almost never become captivated by someone they know well, as an Archives of Sexual Behaviour study on Israeli kibbutz marriages clearly illustrates. It was found that out of 2,769 marriages, none occurred between men and women who had actually grown up together on the kibbutz. And the reason for this? The easy familiarity of having spent their whole lives together was unconsciously translated into a chaste sibling bond instead of a passionate sexual one.

★ Show (off) some leg by hitching your skirt up slightly as you sit down. Or slip on a pair of high-heeled shoes, which enhances the length and shape of your lower limbs. This part of your body exerts an enormous sexual pull for some males. For many men, a long-legged look is dazzling, the reason being that the lengthening of the limbs is a feature of sexual maturity.

★ Your bottom sends out an unmistakable erotic message. Make him want to give it a pinch by wrapping it in a pair of tight-fitting jeans. You'll look like a voluptuous sex goddess.

Get Happy

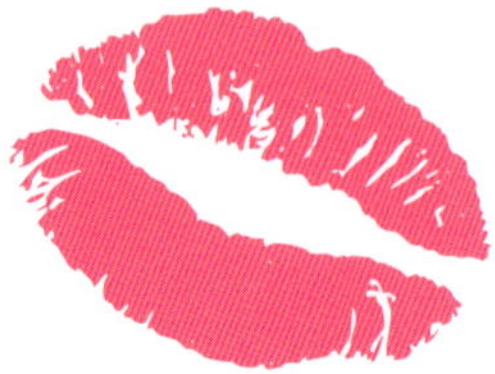

Your mouth gives away your mood. Make yours blissful ...

- ★ Smile only when you mean it. A tight jaw and top lip will seem false and make your face look tension-filled and lopsided. The trick is to learn to relax your face. Practise by scrunching up all your facial muscles as tight as you possibly can for five seconds and then release them. Do this five times, then massage your temples.

- ★ Bare your teeth: both men and women tend to give open smiles whenever they're sexually aroused.

- ★ Bite your lower lip as you smile. This is a very provocative move that will make him want to lean over and give you a long, lingering smooch.

- ★ Smile with your mouth and eyes: this is the most friendly 'I'm-nice-to-know' smile there is. Think happy thoughts to get your face to light up. Adding a little laughter to the mix will put your body in a state of arousal similar to when you are sexually turned on and will make you seem more alluring.

- ★ Part your lips slightly when you smile. It'll make you seem alert, expressive and responsive. Susan Sprecher, professor of Sociology at Illinois University, conducted a cross-cultural survey of 1,667 men and women in the USA, Japan and Russia to find out what people look for in a mate. In all three countries, animation was a bigger draw than looks when it came to what made him want to get to know you better.

- ★ Giggle, but keep your mouth closed or put one hand over it so the sound is much softer. This is less intense than laughter and lets you subtly say, 'I know intimacy is on the menu, but I'm shy.'

Say it with Your Body

Try some of the body moves below to make him feel at ease and connected with you.

★ When you greet him, give off a warm aura simply by resting on one foot more than the other, letting your hip jut out a bit with your hands on the small of your back.

★ As you talk with him, point your knees, feet, hands, shoulders or whole body towards him – it's a subtle way of saying that you aren't complete strangers anymore.

★ Women, more than men, shrink into their spaces by subconsciously tightening their bodies. To avoid this, open your body to him. Open your hands instead of clenching them into fists. Don't fold them in a tight hand grasp; tent the fingertips instead, and rather than sitting with your hands tightly folded, drape them loosely over the arms of the chair. Bonus: the open body represents sexy power (a closed body symbolizes weakness, insecurity or hostility).

★ Affectionate touching tells a guy that you wouldn't mind touching him more in private. If he says something witty, squeeze his forearm gently and laugh. If you want to go to the ladies' room, put your hand on his shoulder and say, 'I'll be right back.'

★ Copy him. When two people become captivated with each other, they begin to subtly and unconsciously mimic each other's postures and gestures within 5 to 50 seconds. Eventually, even breathing and heartbeats become synchronized. Called 'mirroring', it's a learned habit left over from infancy when the newborn mimics its body movements with the rhythmic patterns of whatever voice is speaking to it. You can consciously use mirroring to lure him in by deliberately echoing his movements. But keep it down to less than five gestures or he's going to feel stalked. (If he changes movements every time you start copying him, don't expect him to call you again.)

★ Sitting up with straight, yet relaxed posture shows that you're having a good time and are interested in what he has to say.

When You Only Have 30 Hours

Enchant him, tempt him, tease him. Any guy will tell you that it's the little gestures that achieve BIG results. Best of all, when you have time on your hands, you can s-l-o-w-l-y blaze a sizzling impression on his radar. Check out these can't-resist-you tricks and dazzle the man you desire. Use them on him and in no time at all, he'll be drawn to you like a moth to a flame.

Unexpected Aphrodisiacs

Not-so-obvious ploys will make him stick around.

★ Hum 'Ode to Joy'. An Indiana University study of 239 students reveals that our musical tastes can influence how hot we think someone is, and men are more attracted to women with a taste for classical music. They're still trying to work out why, but in the meantime, pump up the volume!

★ Eat raw mushrooms: the odour is reminiscent of sex. Or just eat in front of him. A New York University survey discovered that most guys think that a woman who picks at her food is a total turn-off (not to mention scary – it's no secret that the most mild-mannered person will turn into an irritable monster when they are food-deprived). Having a healthy appetite makes them think you are going to be a sensuous lover.

★ Practise listening. Studies by language psychologist Deborah Tannen have found that women tend to interrupt more than men, making guys feel like they're not really being listened to. Keeping a little bit silent while you consider what he's saying will make you stand out because you're listening to him. And that will make him want to continue the conversation – over dinner, perhaps?

★ Scare yourselves sexy. Invite the object of your desire to a horror movie or for a ride on a roller-coaster. A Canadian study found that there's evidence that emotional arousal, including experiences that involve fear, triggers off sexual attraction. Research subjects who were either warned of imminent electric shock, scared to death on high, wobbly bridges or told of grotesque mutilations all tested higher for intensity of romantic passion. So did those who ran on the spot for two minutes, were severely embarrassed, or listened to a Steve Martin comedy routine.

Flirty Foreplay

Reduce an otherwise evolved man to a drooling, panting fool.

★ Say his name to fan the flame. Called 'anchoring', the technique of saying his name three times while talking to him will connect him to you. Strengthen the bond between you physically by lightly touching his arm or hand when you repeat his moniker.

★ Use a nickname. According to a study by University of California–Los Angeles psychologist Albert Mehrabian, giving him your own private handle is a quick shortcut to making him feel up-close-and-personal with you.

Pump Up the Passion

The sweet art of seduction is learning how to say, 'Come and get me' without making him feel stalked.

★ Check out the material at work. Most people select a job based on such factors as salary, status and enjoyment. But according to a study of 3,000 singles conducted by Pennsylvania State researchers, about 10 per cent of all love affairs begin on the job. In another survey conducted by several temp agencies, about 2,000 career women claimed that a romance between colleagues is four times more likely to last than an affair between people who meet outside the workplace.

★ Pay a lot of attention to his friends. This triggers off a sense of rivalry in the guy you're after, forcing him to find a way into the conversation and exclude his buddy (never underestimate the competitiveness between men).

★ Along the same lines, get a fake date. If you know a great-looking male friend, by all means show him off. According to research on jealousy conducted by psychologist David Buss, PhD, there are few things more attractive to a man than the fact that other men are attracted to you. In one study, when people were asked to judge women based on photographs of them with 'spouses' of differing attractiveness, unattractive women paired off with good-looking men were routinely rated most favourably in terms of status.

★ Compete with him. Challenge him to a game of tennis and bust his balls. According to a study by John Jay College of Criminal Justice, women who don't hold back their killer instinct are seen as more attractive than those who act in a more demure fashion.

★ Cast a spell over him by throwing pink rose petals (they'll make him want to have sex) and fresh orange peel (for enticement) in your handbag or pocket. Lighting a pink candle before meeting up with him and visualizing how you want him to see you (as a sexy vixen, of course) will also influence his attitude.

Grab Hold of Him

Ways to touch him to let him know you want him – NOW!

★ If you like him and you know it, clap your hands. The truth is, we're more likely to be attracted to someone who is obviously attracted to us. This give-and-take element was confirmed in a University of California study of passion influences, where the perception of being liked ranked just as high as the presence of sex appeal in the potential partner.

★ Flex and he'll think sex. Gestures exposing vulnerable areas such as the underside of your arms, sometimes while fondling a glass or keys, or running a fingertip along the arm of a table tell a man you are ready to expose yourself to him.

★ Remind him of what's beneath your clothes. Dangle a shoe off your bare toe or let the sleeve of your top slip off your shoulder so you're just a little more bare than he expects. One of the greatest turn-ons of all is imagining the parts of another person's body that you can't see. Showing him a little skin, even if it's not the most risqué spot, will be a hint of things to come ... if he plays his cards right.

★ Scientists have observed that people tend to clasp their hands behind their head, elbows pointed skywards and armpits wafting outwards when they want to send out an arousal signal. It's a way of saying, 'Look at me. Listen to me. Smell me. I'm sexy.' (And who's going to argue with a couple of loaded armpits?)

★ Give him a little smooch. A Georgia Tech University study revealed that the sebaceous glands found all over the body act as a sort of bonding agent. When two people ingest each other's sebum, usually through a kiss, they become 'addicted' to each other's chemicals, making them want to couple up to maintain the warm, cuddly feelings all the time.

★ Give him an orgasm. A University of Manchester study indicates that when a person collapses in a joyful heap of contractual ripples, their brain levels of oxytocin, a sort of hormonal superglue, rise, making them feel more attracted and attached to their lover. Unfortunately, it doesn't work the other way around – the researchers found that the degree of romantic attachment had no effect on orgasm.

★ Caressing his head and face has a similar effect (but isn't as much fun!).

★ Leave him guessing. Firmly clasp both your arms around his waist for no more than a few seconds. Then leave him to work out whether that embrace was 'sisterly' or not.

Chapter 2

Things Women Should Know About Men

His Brain

If you're anything like the average female, you sometimes have doubts about what planet men come from: Is he for real? Do all guys act this way? What is he THINKING?

Even though men and women both spend nine months in the womb, have 26 vertebrae in our spines and the same neurochemical pathways in our brains, we spend most of our years without any real understanding of what's actually going on in the other's brain.

Well, you can stop head-scratching (and ruining your 'do). Here's your field guide to the male species. This should settle once and for all why someone who pees differently is so different in every other way as well.

Caution: Don't read the following while eating. This unparalleled peek into the male mind may just make your jaw drop.

Why Can't a Man Be More Like a Woman?

Proof that Mother Nature favours her own sex.

★ Blahblahblah commitment. Blahblahblah cuddling. Blahblahblah seat up. This is what he hears when you talk. Evolutionary studies have found that the male hearing system isn't as fine-tuned as the female's (something to do with meat hunting being more important than baby nurturing). Hence, cut him some slack when he says he didn't hear you. He probably didn't.

★ From about age 12 to 30, all men can think about is getting sex. That's because they're biologically driven to spread genes to as many babes as possible to ensure the survival of their DNA. Which explains why men are also so easy.

- ★ Men and women don't use their brains in the same way. In general, men can only use either their left-brain language skills or their right-brain problem-solving skills, while women can use both at the same time. Which means that if he's talking, he's not thinking and if he's thinking, he's not talking.

- ★ Why does he leave the toilet seat up, practically guaranteeing you'll find yourself hip-deep in toilet water at 3 am? It's all about power, say psychologists who study this sort of thing. It's his way of saying, 'Why is what you want more important than what I want?' (Er, because what a woman wants is more logical, perhaps?)

- ★ On the same theme, his sheets are grimy, not because he has a male 'gross' gene, but because of biology. Men have a weaker sense of smell and their skin isn't as sensitive as women's. So they aren't likely to notice (until live things are thriving) that they're snoozing on stinky sheets.

- ★ The average male is potty-trained by the age of three. So what's with the puddle on the floor? It turns out that peeing straight isn't as easy as it looks. The penis is a dual-purpose machine and many things – including sex – can create a blockage in the pipeline. And drips around the toilet.

- ★ The Y-chromosome set's rabid channel surfing could have something to do with brain degeneration. According to a study conducted at the University of Pennsylvania Medical Center, men lose brain tissue three times faster than women, with some of the largest losses in the parts that control attention span (explaining why he doesn't remember your anniversary, even after you've reminded him 623 times).

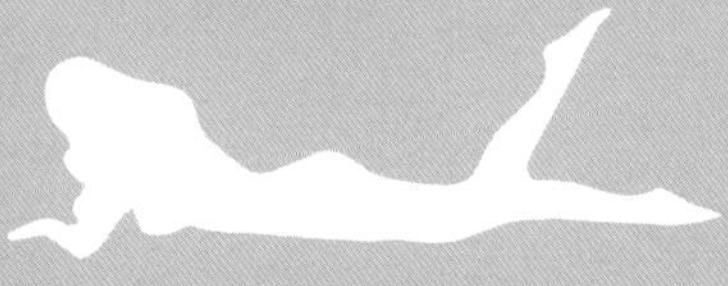

Men Rule!

Yes, men need remedial emotional tutoring. But that doesn't mean women still can't learn a few useful lessons about life from them. Here are four.

1 He can drive. In general, men have a better sense of spatial relations and can judge distances better than women. That's why they tend to do well at things like geometry, figuring out computer games and tail-gating the car in front of them. In other words, he really is more in control than he seems (sometimes, anyway).

2 He understands what's restricted information. Surveys have found that it's WOMEN – not men – who dish the dirt. He'll never reveal what a great girlfriend he has because deep down he's afraid his friends might go after her (see tip 3). So men stick solely with general reports when with their friends – 'She has brown hair' – whereas women will detail everything down to the freckle on his penis.

3 He knows how to compete – particularly with another man over a woman. Men have a severe need to succeed and, once again, biology is to blame. In the face of competition, a man's testosterone level soars, making him more willing to take risks. While this overdrive can be annoying, you may not want to discourage it. According to a study conducted at Pennsylvania State University, testosterone levels of winners stay high post-battle. So if he's lucky, you may get lucky too.

4 The same insensitivity that makes it difficult for him to read people keeps men in good stead for cutting their losses when a relationship isn't working rather than making futile attempts to work things out (hmmm – like anyone you know?).

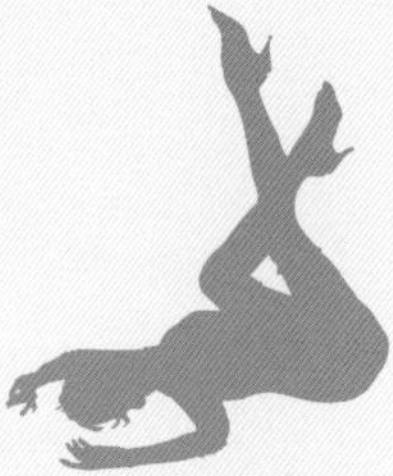

Loser-Proof Your Life

Is he a relationship in the making or the breaking? Checking out his habits is one sure way to know you're not giving your heart to a 'going-nowhere' kind of a guy.

★ Go shopping with him. Watch how he orders in a restaurant. If he um's and ah's between the red and blue T-shirt or always dithers over this choice of drink, he'll probably buckle under the weight of making any decision – including whether he wants a full-time girlfriend or a casual relationship.

★ Find out how many notches he has on his bed-post. A study in the *Journal of Personality and Social Psychology* states that the more a guy sleeps around, the more likely his character type falls under the heading 'Creep'.

Guaranteed orgasms or guaranteed relationship?
Here are five signs he'd be great to Sleep with / Live with:

1 He never makes you hurry up/He never makes you wait.

2 He makes big delicious takes-forever-to-clean-up meals/He scrubs all the pans.

3 He lets you set the pace when you walk/When you start to do something – pour the coffee, pay for the drinks – he often says it's his turn.

4 Seeing him makes your pulse race/Seeing him puts you in a good mood.

5 You're on the same wavelength about condoms, where your hot spots are and a threesome with your best friend/You're on the same wavelength about fidelity, commitment and the future.

10 Big Fat Lies About Men

You can be so wrong about him. Here's what he REALLY thinks.

1 OK, all you cynical, jaded, been-there, done-that, heard-that-line, fell-for-it-anyway, how-could-I-have-been-so-stupid, men-are-the-scum-of-the-earth babes out there. It turns out men aren't the hound dogs we think they are. When a University of Chicago survey asked men what would make them happy, relationship, marriage and family topped the list while sex came near the bottom. Maybe that's because marriage is better for him than it is for you – men make more money, live longer, are happier and have healthier, more and better sex when married than women, according to National Health and Social Life survey of 13,000 adults.

2 Men don't fear intimacy with women. What they fear is intimacy with the WRONG woman. Men, in fact, seek marriage in GREATER numbers than women, and very few remain lifelong bachelors: 94 per cent of males wed at some point in their lives – and, once a man tries marriage, he's hooked. Divorced and widowed men remarry in greater numbers.

3 Yes, he may be more LIKELY to cheat, but a Gallup Poll has uncovered a virtual epidemic of fidelity: 89 per cent of husbands report the only woman they do the wild thang with is their wife. As heartening are the results of a Virginia Slims American Women's Opinion Poll in which more than 75 per cent of the 1,000 men surveyed thought fidelity was more important to a good marriage than a satisfying sexual relationship, financial security or having children.

4 You may think that men's body image issues begin and end with penis size. Wrong. The fact is, 94 per cent of men would like to change some aspect of their physical appearance. And men who think their biceps aren't beefy enough endure the same feelings of inadequacy and depression as women who think their thighs are too thick (see page 56 for more on what he fears body-wise).

5 Just because he's throwing darts three minutes after breaking up with you, don't think he isn't hurting inside. Research from the University of Michigan found that it actually takes men about three times longer to get over a break up than women, but it usually hits them much later. And they recover by keeping busy. Also, although men don't cry so easily after a break-up, they do get impotent, suffer from gastrointestinal disorders, drink more, have automobile accidents and are more likely to commit suicide over a failed love affair.

6 You are more to him than his career. Asked which factors contribute most to a happy, satisfied life, nearly 2,000 men participating in the *Playboy* Report on American Men ranked love second only to health. Work came an unimpressive fifth. But the way men express their love is by providing for their family.

7 Sure, men would LIKE to have sex seven times in one day – but only once in their lives, so they can talk about it forever. Otherwise, most are happy to call it a night after one or two body blast-offs.

8 If one gender had to be labelled starry-eyed romance junkies, it would be the males. They fall in love faster and more often than females. Researchers have found that men are more likely than women to fall deeply in love by the fourth date, be the first to utter 'I love you', believe that true love lasts forever and can overcome all obstacles, and are less likely to end the relationship. Awww.

9 Men are not breast-obsessed. Sure, they like them – a lot. But they don't need triple-letter sizes. When young men were asked to rate front-view line drawings of female physiques for attractiveness in an Archives of Sexual Behavior study, ratings were unaffected by breast size.

10 Men get soppy. But not over *The English Patient*. Sit with him when his favourite team loses, however, and you'll see him weep furiously.

Psych Him Out

Sneaky tactics that make him want what you want – to stay with you.

★ Always be ready to leave. Men thrive on competition and knowing you aren't totally committed cranks him up a gear.

★ If you're looking for a long-term relationship, keep your party dress on until he dials again. Studies show that while the average man will have sex on a first date in a heartbeat, he doesn't want to get involved with a woman willing to sleep with him on the first date because he thinks she's doing this with other men.

★ Bake him a pumpkin pie. Apparently this scent (along with lavender, black liquorice and doughnuts) spikes penile blood flow, according to a Chicago's Smell & Taste Treatment and Research Foundation study.

★ Make it thigh-high and lacy. According to one survey, lingerie ranked way over toys, games and sharing fantasies as the average male's favourite erotic aid.

★ Get ahead. According to a University of Utah study, men are 50 per cent more likely to respond to a personal ad where the woman describes herself as ambitious rather than attractive or slim.

★ Go on the Pill (once you know he's safe). The reality is that he doesn't care about using condoms because he isn't as afraid of AIDS, STDs and pregnancy as you are. And research backs him up. Women are TWO TIMES more likely to be infected through sex with a man who's infected than a man would be through sleeping with a woman who's infected.

★ Say you'd rather stay at home tonight. Researchers at the University of Illinois found that men are basically nesters, happiest at home, even while doing the chores. (Women are more likely to go into a joy trance away from *la casa*.) The reason? He feels more in control in his own surroundings, giving him home-court advantage.

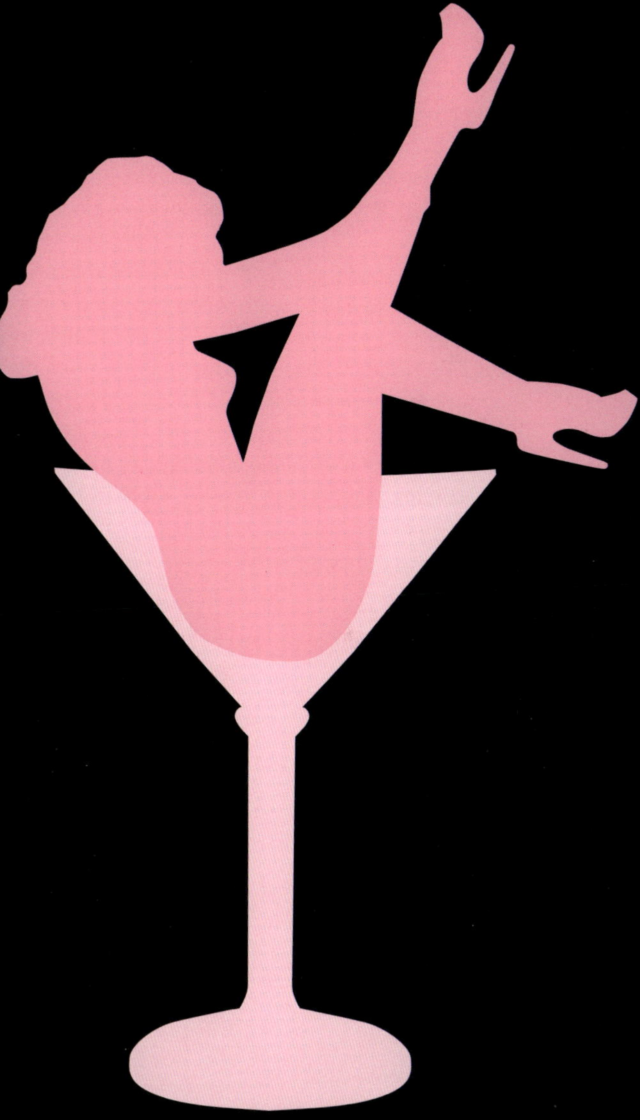

His Heart

As a gender, men have a lot to answer for. Not just warfare, topless models and Arnold Schwarzenegger, but all their pitiable excuses, the total selfishness, the strategic hot-and-cold attitude – all quiet little ways of treating a relationship as anything other than the delicate little soufflé it is.

However, splicing jokes aside, it's clear that the one thing ALL men want is a relationship (or at least say they do when you get them alone after a few beers and a particularly bad day). They just don't want to initiate it, work at it, talk about it or think about it. The reality is, men are not trying to avoid ALL women – they're trying to avoid all but one. The One.

To understand what makes a man see a woman as the one he wants to marry and other insights into his true desires, read on.

Man Watching

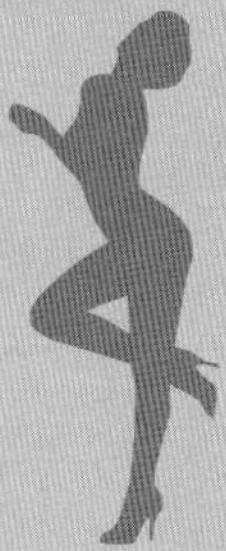

How well do you pick up the silent signals a man sends?

When a guy says he'll call you, it's hard to tell if he means it (see page 49 for more on this), but something in the way he moves can provide a few clues:

- He looks at you: Your bust, that is. And then he makes contact with your eyes.
- He ignores you: No guy actively avoids female attention, unless he's already enjoyed yours and decided not to go there again. So this is his pathetic way of trying to make you think he's cool as opposed to desperate.
- He stands so close to you that you know what he had for breakfast: He's trying to tell you that he's attracted to you, but in a way that suggests he may be telling you what to wear and who you can hang out with in the future.
- He thrusts his chest at you: This is an instinctive move all males make to attract a mate – in short, he wants you.
- He grooms himself, patting his hair, adjusting his clothes, tugging his chin: He's saying 'Look at me! Look at me! Look at me!'
- He's rubbing his own arm or chest: He's thinking, Me, Tarzan; You, Jane'.
- He touches your arm: He feels touchy-feely towards you – get ready for a kiss.
- He's sitting with legs wide open: He's an alpha-male, splaying what he's got and saying, 'Come and get it!'

You're clearly giving him the Yes signal but he still doesn't make a move (dammit!). The reason is that he doesn't have a clue. The way you run your fingers through your hair might mean you want him to kiss you like you've never been kissed before or it might mean your scalp is itchy. Who knows? He certainly doesn't. So, not to put too fine a point on it, if you want him, take him. He won't mind.

Accessorize!

He may be tall, cuter than Brad Pitt, hold a job, have ready cash and practically smell of sex, but STILL be a commitment-phobic two-timing jerk. Pay attention to his trimmings – according to psychologists, things like his favourite colour and snack are what give away his inner bloke.

HE DRESSES …

- ♥ Bottom Up (knickers, socks, trousers, shoes, shirt, tie): Well-grounded – he'll always pay the rent and keep his promises.
- ♥ Top Down (shirt, tie, knickers, trousers, socks, shoes): Hates details. Frequently misplaces keys and forgets to call. But he'll blow his rent on sexy lingerie for you.
- ♥ Varies: Changeable – might not be dependable.

HIS SNACK ATTACKS …

- ♥ Crisps: A social butterfly. Enjoy the ride but you'll need patience to net him.
- ♥ Candy: Still a kid at heart. Sounds like fun …until you have to pay all the bills yet again because he's spent his salary on boy toys.
- ♥ Sandwiches: Tough and determined, he'll work hard to please you.
- ♥ Chocolate: Since it contains chemicals that bring on a natural high, his craving could signal a need for instant gratification – which won't satisfy your need for commitment.

HIS OUTER BEAST …

- ♥ German Shepherd-type Dog: A crotch sniffer.
- ♥ Labrador-type Dog: Friendly and fun, but needs lots of exercise.
- ♥ Corgi-type Dog: Annoyingly smart but good at respecting space.
- ♥ Rottweiler-type Dog: Protective jealous type – potential abuser.
- ♥ Persian Cat: Hard to please and a bit lazy.
- ♥ Short-Haired Cat: Self-confident.
- ♥ Bird/Fish/Any Reptile: Will back off as soon as it seems you're getting close.
- ♥ Rodent: A secret trainspotter.
- ♥ Menagerie: Easy-going, nurturing and social, but also has lots of demands on his attention.

His Pet Girlfriend Peeves

Do these and he'll behave like a cornered rat – bolting at the first opportunity.

1 Talk dirty – about an ex. When you're in love, the desire to open the book to your life is intoxicating. Just remember: men are often insecure sexually (see page 58) and hearing you've done it all with some other guy can be unsettling. A man's checklist of need-to-know information is short: 'Do you have an STD? Are you on trial for a violent crime? Are you married?' Beyond that, he just doesn't wanna know.

2 Share too much: He doesn't want you to dish all to your friends, no matter how adorable it was that he cried when his team won the championship. (On the other hand, any tales of his amazing stud abilities are fine for general broadcast.)

3 Push his head down during sex. He'll get there when he gets there. And he WILL get there. Recent polls reveal that muff diving is a top guy activity (right after boning).

4 Put him through endless chat on the phone. There's only one type of conversation he gets into – it's called phone sex.

5 Discuss the future. You're together – isn't that enough? Do you have to talk about it all the time? (If you let the 'F' word slip, don't worry – read pages 40–1).

Why Men Stay

What makes a man get down on bended knee?

★ You're like the girl next door. Men divide women into two categories – those you screw and those you marry. He likes wild and crazy – but not to spend the rest of his life with.

★ According to studies, when men are just on the trawl, they seek the Pamela Anderson formula of sexiness. But when they're looking for someone to marry, it's more likely to be someone who is beautiful in their own mind.

★ You caught him at the right 'Tom' moment. There are Toms (as in Cruise) and there are Toms (as in Hanks). One is forever a boy; the other, though boyish, is definitely a man – a man who realizes he wants to marry, have children and settle down.

★ Keep him guessing. The number one male fantasy is sex with lots of women. So when you constantly surprise him, he never has a chance to get bored. However, since there are only so many sexual positions, scents, camisoles, lipsticks, breath-freshener tricks and so on in the universe, spread them out over a chunk of time to keep him interested.

His Cheating Heart

What makes a guy roam outside his home turf?

A worldwide study of over 37 different cultures established what you knew all along – men cheat more than women. The dilemma: they also want to marry a woman with little sexual experience. The reason: they have a biological imperative to spread their own genes but don't want to end up supporting some other bloke's little genes. According to research on an average cheat's profile, here's how to know for sure if you suspect yours is not the only station he is servicing:

- He refuses to consider living together, even though you spend all your time together.
- He swept you off your feet (he's a serial romantic).
- He's over-detailed when explaining where he's been / who with and for how long (he's getting his story straight).
- He consistently heads straight for the bathroom before you've even kissed him hello (he's removing evidence).
- He develops an incredible new sexual technique (this might make it almost worth it).

According to a University of Indiana study, men are more likely to stray more when:

- There's a baby in the house (not him).
- Someone else gets ahead of him career-wise (he thinks, 'I'm a loser').
- YOU get ahead of him career-wise (he thinks, 'I'm a wussy loser').
- He has a big win (he thinks he's so cool that everyone loves him and wants him).
- He starts losing his hair – or anything else that reminds him he's getting older, fatter, uglier.
- He falls in love (it's his cute way of saying he really cares about you – so much that it scares him right into another woman's arms).
- A woman makes it clear she wants him.
- He suspects you're cheating.

His Tongue

There's an old joke about a wife who nags her husband, 'Tell me how you feel'. Finally, the husband blurts, 'I feel … I feel … like watching television'.

The awful truth is, most men have no idea how they feel at any given time. Studies show that men use language to establish difference, separateness and independence (exactly the opposite of women, who talk to connect). So demanding that he talk to you is guaranteed to make him squirm and start rambling about whether new Cheerios really are improved.

Here are the answers and explanations to his biggest verbal 'Huhs?' (you'll be speaking like a native in no time).

Man-Speak

An at-a-glance guide to his love talk.

A slew of research has established that men and women use language in different ways. For women, talk is the glue that holds relationships together. To men, conversation is a means, not an end. They don't even like talking to each other that much – two guys can watch a game in silence for four hours and walk away feeling they've bonded. When men do use words, it's primarily doublespeak to stay on top. Here's how to make sense of the favourite phrases he uses for different stages of your union.

WHEN YOU'RE DATING

HE SAYS: So maybe we could get together or something?
HE MEANS: I think you're really hot and want to ask you out, but I'm too chicken to say so.

HE SAYS: Nothing about seeing you again.
HE MEANS: His mojo wasn't rising.

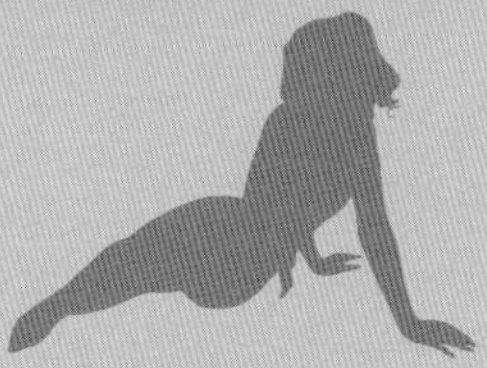

HE SAYS: You're a really good person.
HE MEANS: You'll never see him again.

HE SAYS: Let's be friends.
HE MEANS: You're not my type, but could you set me up with your hot friend?

HE SAYS: I'll call you.
HE MEANS: I really mean to call but I'm scared you'll say yes, we'll go out, and it will be a letdown. Or worse, what if it's not? Do I want to go through all the hassle of dating? Get married? Have kids? Aaahhhh!

HE SAYS: We're dating.
HE MEANS: We've spent at least five nights together, at least one of which has ended in sexual contact. But in no way are we exclusive.

HE SAYS: We're seeing each other.
HE MEANS: It's down to you and one other woman.

HE SAYS: I think we should date exclusively.
HE MEANS: I'm scared that if I don't make things more permanent, you'll date someone else.

WHEN HE WANTS SEX
HE SAYS: This is our third date, isn't it?
HE SAYS: Is it warm out or just me?
HE SAYS: What time do you go to work in the morning?
HE SAYS: You think it's true what they say about oysters?
HE MEANS: I WANT SEX

HE SAYS (IN THE MIDDLE OF A GREAT ORGASM): I love you.
HE MEANS: I love that incredible thing you are doing with your finger/tongue/body right now.

HE SAYS (IMMEDIATELY AFTER MAKING LOVE): It'll be great to show you the house I grew up in (or anything else that smacks of the future).
HE MEANS: Are you thinking about your ex and how much better he was than me?

HE SAYS: We haven't spoken for ages and I've been thinking about you.
HE MEANS: I haven't gotten laid in almost three months.

HE SAYS: I'm not looking to get serious.
HE MEANS: I just want a little nookie.

HE SAYS: How many guys have you been with?
HE MEANS: I'm the best, right?

WHEN YOU'RE A COUPLE

HE SAYS: I really like you.
HE MEANS: I think I am falling in love but if I say that word, there is no going back.

HE SAYS (IN MIDDLE OF A DATE): It'll be great to show you the house I grew up in (or anything else that smacks of the future).
HE MEANS: See above.

HE SAYS: 'Girlfriend' and he's not doing a Ru Paul imitation.
HE MEANS: You've made him breakfast, he fixed your car and his buddies aren't allowed to come on to you.

HE SAYS: Nothing's wrong. I'm fine.
HE MEANS: God, I know you want to talk about my day and all my inter-relationships with my colleagues and boss, and the guy who drives my bus, but I am home now and I just want to drink ten beers, eat a bag of chips for dinner and zone out.

HE SAYS: Maybe we need to slow down.
HE MEANS: Maybe you need to slow down.

HE SAYS: I don't know what I want.
HE MEANS: I don't want you.

HE SAYS: I need some space.
HE MEANS: I'm about this close to dumping you but I haven't worked up the nerve yet.

HE SAYS: You're an amazing woman.
HE MEANS: You're an amazing woman.

HE SAYS: I love you.
HE MEANS: You make me incredible happy whenever we are together. I think you may be The One.

As noted in the beginning of the chapter, men don't always hear everything you're saying. Which means he's not always getting your message.

YOU SAY (AFTER BEING INTRODUCED): Do you know this band?
HE HEARS: I want you now.

YOU SAY: What do you do?
HE HEARS: Are you making enough money to be marriage material?

YOU SAY: My ex is a crazy stalker who won't stop calling me. He scares me.
HE HEARS: I'm still in love with my ex.

YOU SAY: What are we doing Saturday night?
HE HEARS: I want all your time for the rest of your life.

YOU SAY (AFTER MAKING LOVE): That was really nice.
HE HEARS: That was the best sex of my life. Let's do it again!

Top Lies Men Tell Women

- ★ But I TRIED to call.
- ★ I didn't get the message.
- ★ I didn't notice what she looked like.
- ★ Sex isn't the most important thing.
- ★ I'll be careful.
- ★ We'll talk about it later.
- ★ I'm not mad.
- ★ I could fall in love with you in a minute (wait a minute and ask him how he feels now).

Talking His Talk

How to talk to a man so he understands you.

Men can only take directions one at a time. So if you want him to go into the kitchen and get you a cup of tea, make it a two-part request (this also applies to when you are in bed with him).

When men bother to use words, it's to inspire action (whereas women communicate to bond). So if a guy insults another guy, he automatically thinks he wants to fight. And if you say you like his shirt, he thinks, 'Cool – she wants to jump my bones!'

University of Houston psychologists investigating why men keep things bottled up found it was to maintain power in a relationship – when they don't talk, their partner is left guessing. You do the same and he'll be putty in your hands.

Men don't want to talk about the relationship. They just want to do it (in his mind, if he didn't love you, he'd leave). Here's how he thinks: 'If we need to talk about the relationship, it must be broken. If it's broken, it means it's doomed. I'm outta here.'

A man will say, 'I'm fine', even when being tortured by Zulu warriors. It's in his nature not to reveal weakness because that betrays vulnerability, which comes off as lack of status, according to research by evolutionary psychologist David Buss. In short, he's worried you'll think he's a weed if he can't solve his problems without his Superwoman girlfriend coming to his aid.

There are certain words his tongue seem to trip over – like 'girlfriend', 'love' and 'commitment'. But since men are action-driven, what he does is more important than what he says. You know your man really loves you if he:

- ♥ Lets you drive his car.
- ♥ Assumes you're spending the weekend together.
- ♥ Introduces you to his friends.
- ♥ Stops wearing his 'If you're not wasted, the day is' T-shirt, because he knows you hate it.
- ♥ Calls for absolutely no reason.
- ♥ Wants to talk after sex.

Here's what he really doesn't want to ever hear from you (and probably won't hear anyway):

- ♥ Honey, we have to talk. No, YOU have to talk – and talk and talk and talk.
- ♥ What are you thinking about? His feelings, like his answers, will be simple. So if you are lying in post-coital comfort and he answers, 'Pizza', he really means he is thinking about pizza and not that you have skin that resembles pizza or you look like you've eaten one too many pies in your life.
- ♥ Do you think that girl is pretty? He thinks that if he even hesitates to say no, it will kill his chances of sex that night – or any other night.
- ♥ I want to get married. He already assumes this is what you want, he just doesn't want to hear it. So you only have to notify him if this is NOT the case.
- ♥ How do I look – honestly? Honestly, you look wonderful to him. That's why he's with you.

His Private Parts

What's his world view? Depends. Is he: About to have an orgasm? In the midst of having one? Just finished having one?

If it sometimes seems that a man thinks with his penis, it's because he does. Hormones dictate that he has one biological function: to deposit sperm. In anyone, any time, anywhere. In short, the essential distinction between a man and a woman can be summed up in a single word: testosterone.

Now that you understand his primary driving force, it's time to get a handle on that holiest of appliances: his genitals. To be honest, most women don't have a clue as to what's going on down there. You know men pee, zip, tuck, scratch and, every once in a lucky while (they think), they spelunk – and sometimes it seems all at once. But don't worry. There's nothing to programme, no wires to splice. Not a shred of assembly is required. So roll up your sleeves, and turn down the sheets.

Below the Belt

A do-it-yourselfer's guide to the worldwide family of penis owners.

A man with a big nose just has a big nose. Actually, the size of his tool depends on his background rather than the size of any other part of his anatomy. Here's the score, according to a study published by the Charles Darwin Research Institute:

BLACK MEN: 16 to 20 cm (6¼ to 7⅞ in) long and 5 cm (2 in) diameter when erect.
WHITE MEN: 14 to 15 cm (5½ to 5⅞ in) long and 3.3 to 4 cm (1⅜ to 1⅝ in) diameter when erect.
ASIAN MEN: 10 to 14 cm (4 to 5½ in) long and 3.2 cm (1¼ in) diameter when erect.

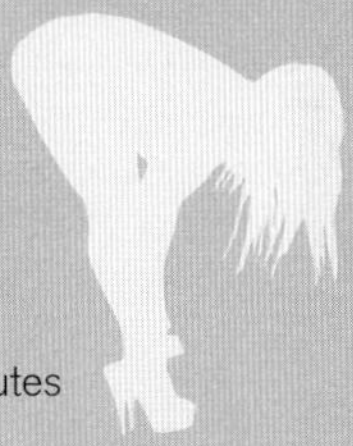

★ Get out your stopwatch. Kinsey studies found that it generally takes a twentysomething three to five minutes to stand to attention (this reaction time doubles with age).

★ Cool your heels (and other body parts). After orgasm, a man enters a refractory or down period where he has to wait anywhere from five minutes (in his teens) to a day (if he's 50+) until the next stiffy comes along.

★ Read washing instructions. The following can shrink a relaxed penis by 5 cm (2 in) or more: cold weather, chilly baths or showers, sexual activity, illness, exhaustion, excitement (nonsexual). Seems it's a protective mechanism. His penis needs a nice warm environment or else it instinctively goes into hiding.

Three things even he doesn't know about his sperm:

1 His sperm has legs. It can live for 5 to 7 days inside you.
2 It would take a sperm 30 minutes to travel across this page.
3 A teaspoon of ejaculate can contain more than 600 million sperm (although this is enough to populate the UK ten times over, there's only a 15 per cent chance that one of them will score a direct hit). The average amount of semen per ejaculation increases if he downs a few beers, hasn't had sex since Sylvester Stallone had a hit movie and eats zinc and vitamin C.

★ He may not feel your pain, but he feels another guy's. The one sure place a man hurts is his groin. The area is so chockablock full of ultrasensitive nerve endings that they even respond when someone gets a poke in the privates.

★ He gets blue when he doesn't have sex. When a man is aroused, blood floods not only to the penis but to the entire area. The longer he stays aroused, the longer the blood stays there. Newer blood is red, but older blood, which has less oxygen, is blue, giving his balls a bluish hue. However, it's not harmful, so don't let him use this as a seduction line.

★ Men as embryos were also women. After testosterone is added, they become boys – but with a few souvenirs left over – such as nipples, a hymen and a vagina masculina.

His Best Friend

His penis made him do it (so don't take it personally).

A recent Kaiser study found that 59 per cent of single men didn't use a condom the last time they had sex. The top reason: no quickies on the steps (that is, a lack of spontaneity); complaints that wearing a rubber was like eating a steak covered in clingfilm (saranwrap) followed a close second.

If he's a gawker, he may just be following his basic instincts. Men are programmed to respond to visual stimuli like porn, erotic undies and gorgeous babes in order to spread sperm and propagate the species. Which is why the quickest way to a man's groin is through his eyes.

The male member has over 200 different 'official' pet names; the most popular being Mr Happy (he wishes!). Though medical science is still sceptical, men name their penises because they believe the penis has a brain completely separate from their own. How else can they explain why they choose to follow its suggestions on major life choices?

He often has sex with the one he loves. Sex therapists joke that 90 per cent of men masturbate at least once a week and the other 10 per cent are lying about it. Call it McSex – jerking off is quick, convenient and satisfying without G-spot worries.

Don't Touch

What makes a guy lose his lust?

Common sense tells us that a man may not be erect because he's not excited. But impotence – otherwise known in slang as erectile dysfunction – is often separate from lack of sexual desire. In fact, in the under-40s set, it is almost always the result of TOO MUCH desire, which leads to a fear of failure and then to failure itself. (But you knew that already, didn't you?)

No work, no wood. To test the effects of stress on sexual function, researchers had a group of jobless men and a group of employed men watch adult movies. Stress was induced by telling the guys they'd have to talk about their own sexual behaviour and fantasies afterwards to a group of students. When they knew that later they'd have to spill their guts sexually, the jobless men had poorer erections during the videos than the employed men. Conclusion: There must be a better way for the unemployed to see free porn.

University of Houston studies have found that anger makes his desire wane, while anxiety (they used the threat of electric shock!) actually increases the size of his erections (stress could make it go either way). Conclusion: Forget about good make-up sex, get him nervous and stop worrying about stressing him out.

Sexual Cravings

No, lots of instant sex with boatloads of women does NOT top the list.

The turn-on of a woman who gets the sexual ball rolling can hardly be under-estimated (with special bonus points going to those who've tried the greet-him-telling-him-you're-not-wearing-underwear game). Putting his hand somewhere that would get you arrested if you did it in the supermarket goes a long way towards appeasing his secret terror that no matter how deeply attracted he is to you, you won't like him.

Because the penis is where men feel pleasure most intensely, you can never pay too much attention to it – love it, adore it, worship it. And because men are much more visual creatures than women, he doesn't just want to look during sex – he needs to. If you really want to make his tongue hang out, do it with the lights on.

Similarly, let him see himself naked. Researchers had men sit naked in a chair with and without a board covering their laps. They then watched some porno. The ones who didn't wear the board had the firmest erections. The point of all this: Men become more stimulated if they can actually see that they are stimulated.

How to Touch a Naked Man

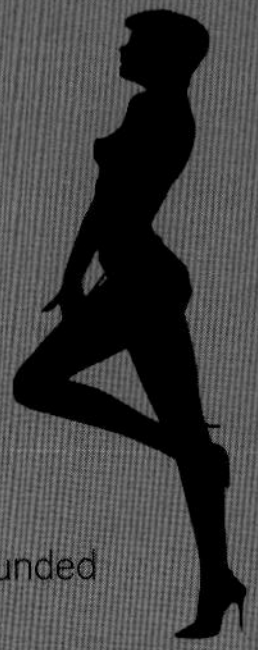

Flip his switch and turn him on.

Your man has his own G-spot. Owing to its location at the base of the penis, a man's erection is more-or-less anchored upon the prostate, a randy nerve-rich gland so sensitive it even secretes fluid during arousal and ejaculation.
BEST MOVE: Slip a well-lubricated finger through the rectum and probe the rounded back wall of the prostrate. When you feel a firm, round, walnut-size lump, gently caress it while stroking his penis.

A man's erection doesn't end at the base of the penis. There's a railroad junction full of nerves in the perineum, that smooth triangle of flesh between the base of his penis and his anus which, when pressed, will send him straight into an orgasmic swoon.
BEST MOVE: Gently rub the spot with the pad of your finger or thumb. (Pressing really hard with one forceful push can actually stop him from peaking, so be careful.)

Stroking his frenulum – the vertical ridge that extends from the tip to the shaft of the penis – will hit his moan zone. Not only are there more nerve endings there, but the skin is also extremely thin.
BEST MOVE: Clenching your pelvic muscles just as he pulls out will give his F-Spot a massage.

Many men are surprised to discover the range and depth of the sensation when you stroke their raphe, the visible line along the centre of the scrotum. They may even end up ejaculating sooner than they (and you) planned.
BEST MOVE: Excite this lust locale by gently running your fingertips along it.

Don't forget his ego – a little stroking goes a long way towards making him relaxed and open to intimacy.
BEST MOVE: Make him feel that you want him.

Can a Man Ever Have Bad Sex?

Five facts about his Big O – this stuff is so secret even he doesn't know it!

1 Timing is everything. In short, when he's about to come, let him go with the flow (unless he's aiming for tip 3). If he blows those final few seconds before ejaculation, his orgasm will be a dud.

2 It may seem as though he can have an orgasm just rubbing against a tree. But it's not that simple. A satisfying experience for a man involves lots of pressure. That's why the hard thrusting at the end of intercourse is so important.

3 He can also have more than one orgasm. In a State University of New York Health Science Center study, men aged 22 to 56 had from three to ten orgasms during extended bouts of sexual stimulation without ejaculation. Their favourite moment: stopping stimulation just at the brink of orgasm, then starting again once they regained control.

4 In men, orgasm and ejaculation are not the same thing. The first is the physical and mental release of sexual tension while the second refers to the release of semen, which can sometimes occur without orgasm. In other words, he can fake it too (and 43 per cent have done so at least once).

5 The real reason men snooze after sex: It seems that oxytocin, a hormone that stimulates women's orgasmic contractions and his erection and ejaculation, also causes drowsiness. But because women's bodies normally contain more of it, they may be less sensitive to its surges. Men, on the other hand, fall into a drunken stupor from it.

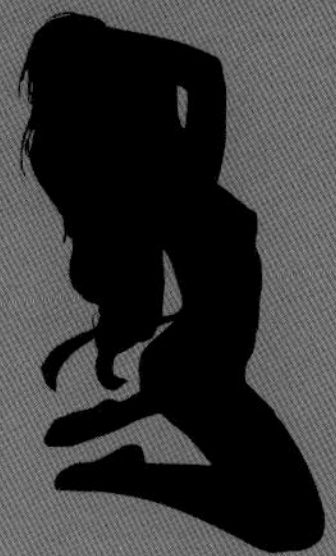

His Hair

Although men may lead you to believe they can handle absolutely anything, the reality is that your average guy has lots of fears. Even the biggest, strongest he-man can turn into a trembling powder-puff of anxiety given the right circumstances.

And nowhere – nowhere – is a man more likely to have a meltdown than in how he relates to you. Men panic when something threatens their sense of self, and most men's self-concept (as you probably guessed) is rooted in their sex life (read: penis). Put another way, guys freak out over anything and everything from asking you out to making whoopee with you. Here are the top fears that plague men (not that they'll ever tell you). Use your knowledge wisely.

Life Concerns

Bottom line: Being a man is a scary business.

★ He's scared of violating the Code of Guys: A man will not appear to be ruled by his girlfriend, his mother, his boss or anything other than his penis for fear of being ousted from the group.

★ He's worried about his thread count: Most men would rather be castrated than go bald. The trouble is that everyone can see his hair all the time, while penises manifest themselves only to a chosen few. No one ever had a thinning penis.

★ He's afraid of you: This can be traced back millions of years to men being awed by things women can do that they can't – menstruate, have children, do more than two things at the same time (if you think men have made any progress after 2.5 million years, try saying 'tampon' in a roomful of guys).

Love Worries

The more he is into you, the more scared he gets.

HIS BIGGEST DATING DOUBTS:

1 Making the first move: Because men are often expected to make the first move, we assume they're used to being turned down. Not so. Whether he's 14 or 34, calling you for a date is like phoning the undertaker to arrange his own funeral. Surveys have found that men feel they're putting their manhood on the line every time they ask you out (a little appreciation on your part goes a long way for him).

2 What to talk about: In his mind, silence equals death. Whenever there's a pause in the conversation he thinks, 'It's over! She's noticed my receding hairline'.

3 Whether to smooch: Go back to tip 1, above.

4 Calling you for a second date: Making a woman wait for the follow-up call is a man's way of gaining back the upper hand. Unfortunately this leaves you in the position of not knowing whether the phone is silent because he doesn't like you, or because he does.

HE'S SCARED OF SETTLING BECAUSE:

1 What if Pamela Anderson calls? No matter how incredible you are (plenty), he's haunted by the possibility of never getting it again.

2 He may like you TOO much. Ergo – he wants nothing more to do with you. This is because he fears a) you won't like him as much; or b) you will, shortly followed by quitting your job, having 16 children, five dogs, demanding a six-bedroom mansion and so on – all of which means he will work for the rest of his life in order to support you.

3 Getting into a committed relationship will tame him. And it will. A Syracuse University study found that testosterone levels are high in single men, decrease in married men and rise in divorced men. This is possibly because single men need to be more aggressive to be able to compete for women, while married men can mellow out because they have the goods and can therefore get on with it.

4 You'll find out that he really does want marriage (although maybe not to you).

5 He will have to start putting the toilet seat down.
6 He's worried you'll cheat on him. Seems it's men who have the real raging hormones. A New Zealand study found that because of his high testosterone levels, he's still prone to jealousy freak-outs and suspicion. So next time he pulls his third-degree act, just tell yourself it must be his time of the month.
7 He's anxious you'll break up with him.
8 He's terrified his mother will like you. Or not like you. Sorry – you can't win this one.

Meet Mr Softee

What pushes his sexual panic buttons?

★ Bulletin: Self-esteem ain't just a girl thing. Crippling as an unreturned phone call … able to fell tall erections with a single 'It's OK, let's just go to sleep' … devastating as the seventeenth mention of the solicitor-rock-climber-gourmet chef at your gym … in truth, it's amazing he's ever able to perform at all. Bringing us to …

★ He has opening-night jitters. Is it big enough? Will it stay up long enough? The reality is that men are so often preoccupied with how they'll appear and perform as sexual partners that they're rarely scrutinizing women as much as women fear they're being scrutinized (in one poll of over 3,000 men, anxiety as to whether he has what it takes to please a woman was the top fear). The possibility that a female he fancies may not want to kiss him, sleep with him, sleep with him a second time or eventually fall in love with him is often enough to make men bail emotionally (explaining why he's uncomfortable and silent the minute after he sleeps with you, even though he is clearly nuts about you).

★ Condoms.

★ Coming too quickly.

★ Impotence.

★ He's worried you'll figure out he doesn't know the way. Men don't ask for directions in bed for the same reason they don't ask for directions in general. Hormones. According to research by evolutionary psychologist Helen Fisher, PhD, communication is linked to the hormone oestrogen. Since men have significantly less oestrogen, they're less verbal and more action-oriented. That means it's up to you to give your honey a helping hand when it comes to locating your hot spots.

★ He thinks he'll never get any again after age 30. According to the University of Chicago's General Social Survey, men have the most sexual intercourse between the ages of 18 and 29. The majority of men in this age-group report bumping bones one or two times a week. After that, the slow, inexorable slide begins. So by age 70, you can expect to be getting lucky only once a month.

★ He's afraid you'll want to cuddle after sex. Let's face it, for men, intercourse culminating with orgasm is the main goal. Everything else is like little paper umbrellas in drinks – fussy and getting in the way of (in this case) sleep.

★ Two words – marathon sex. Guys know women dig tons of foreplay. The problem is, they confuse body caresses with actual penetration and think you want intercourse to last longer than the re-release of *Apocalypse Now*. And if they don't go the distance, they fear they'll be labelled a lame lover and you'll therefore seek out a man blessed with more stamina. Result: Every encounter has him straining to break the world record (put his mind and penis at ease by whispering, 'Don't hold back').

★ According to one survey, most men think women are not fond of the penis. Added to this are his insecurities about size and performance. So a woman who lets him know she likes his best friend is the equivalent of a man saying, 'You are the most wonderful woman I have ever met'.

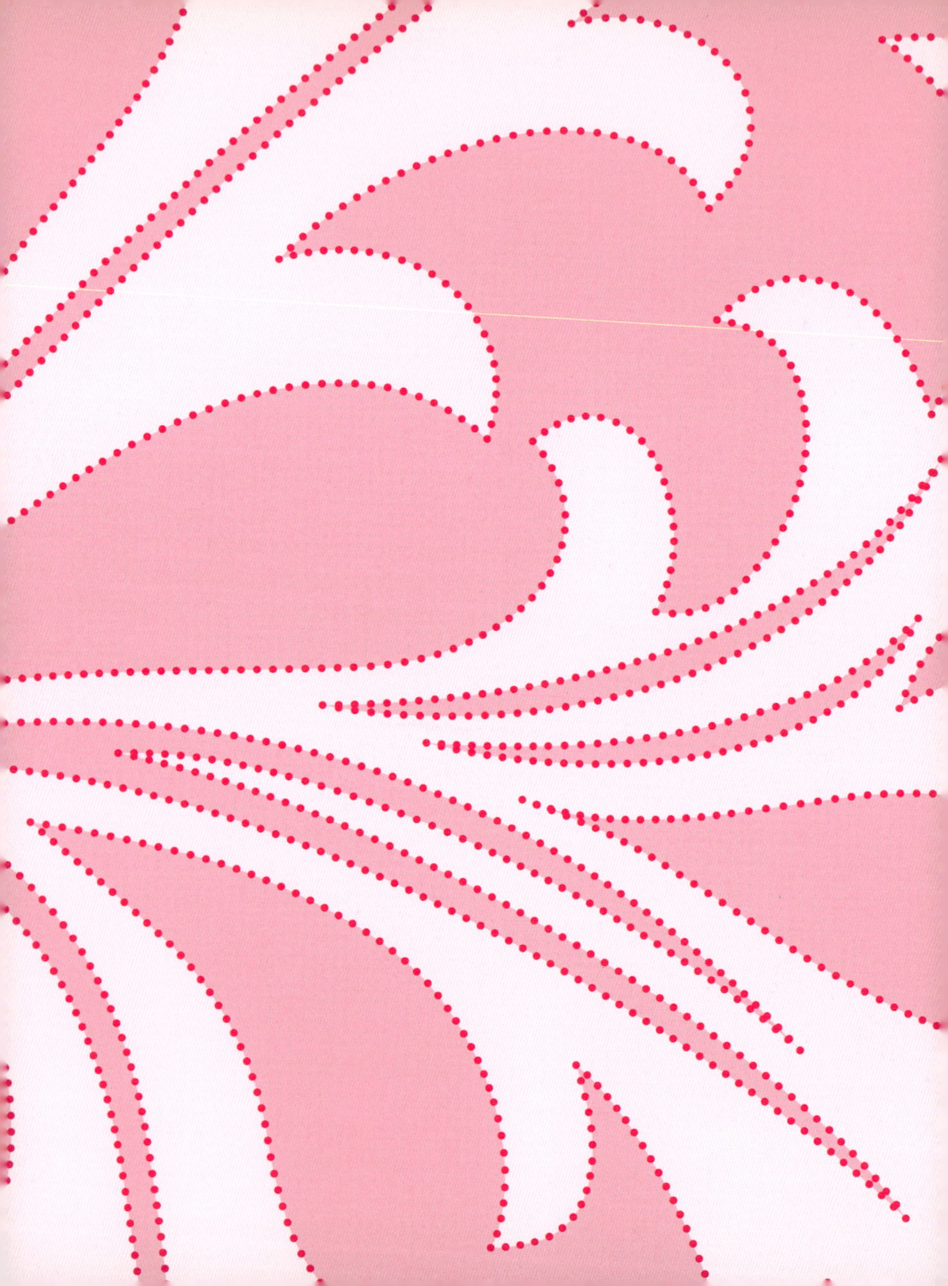

Chapter 3

Sex Positions

RATINGS

To give you some guidelines, some of the following positions have been road-tested and rated as follows:

GETTING IT RIGHT		ORGASMIC POTENTIAL	
✪	Easy peasy.	★	Sweet comfortable screw.
✪✪	Read the directions carefully.	★★	A bit of a body rattler.
✪✪✪	Sexpertise required.	★★★	A real sock roller.

Erotic Sex

In other words, enjoying happy horizontal hula simply for pleasure's sake. Don't just settle for missionary monotony! Whether you're stuck in a sexual rut or just eager for some between-the-sheets experimentation, here's the ultimate guide to positioning yourself (and your partner) for the best sex ever. Let the games begin!

Take Up Your Positions ...

For some triple X-rated twists on the old in and out.

MAN ON TOP (AKA 'MISSIONARY')

THE OLD MOVE: The classic man on top, woman beneath him, face-to-face position. It's great for easy thrusting (him) and creating close, intimate contact between you.

MAKE IT BETTER: Do the knee-chest. Raise your legs so that your knees are pressed to your chest, then drape your legs over his shoulders. He can penetrate you more deeply and give you more friction where you crave it most – on your vaginal lips and clitoris.

✪ ★★

WOMAN ON TOP

THE OLD MOVE: This lets you stay in control and show your stuff. Simply sit on his penis and rotate those hips! Sitting is for sex in slow motion – the angles are all wrong for any sort of energetic thrusting. The man either sits in a chair or cross-legged on the floor, while you sit astride him, usually face to face, although it can work equally well if you face away from him. This position is good for caressing and intimacy.

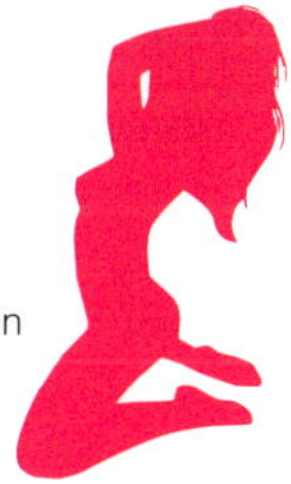

MAKE IT BETTER: Face his toes instead of his head. Then, as you lift yourself up and down, rotate your body in small circles. Tease him by using your vaginal lips to rub his erect penis – tantalize him by degrees until he's squirming. ✪ ✪ ★

STANDING

THE OLD MOVE: Standing is best for quickie trysts, but if he's much taller than you it's difficult to manage as he has to hold you up or you have to stand on a stool so his penis can reach your vagina.

MAKE IT BETTER: Turn around and lean over to give him a delicious view of your derrière. Lift one leg sideways so he can slip inside you without having to twist, then close your legs slightly so he doesn't pop out. His hands can slip around to your clitoris to add a little extra heat. ✪ ✪ ✪ ★★★

SIDE BY SIDE (AKA 'SPOONING')

THE OLD MOVE: Side by side is a lovely cuddly move that's perfect for canoodling. The classic is spooning (lying on your side facing away from him so that he enters you from behind with his arms wrapped around you).

MAKE IT BETTER: Have your lover lie on his back. Then, facing away from him, lower your crotch onto his (your arms should be stretched out behind you to support your weight). He encircles your waist with his legs and grips your thighs. Then you both roll over together onto your sides. He can then thrust gently into you … ✪ ✪ ★★★

REAR ENTRY (AKA 'DOGGIE')

THE OLD MOVE: The classic doggie-style position is a pleasure howler that gives ultra-deep penetration. You kneel on all fours and he slips in from behind …
MAKE IT BETTER: Your partner lies on his back with a pillow beneath his head so he can watch all the action. Facing his feet, you straddle him. Then, placing your hands on the floor first, you back onto his penis. He holds your thighs or buttocks tightly while you thrust up and down the entire length of him. This is doing it doggie your way – you have maximum control while your partner gets to savour every sensation without working up too much sweat. It's a fantastic position for a truly intense G-spot orgasm. ✪ ★★

Push Your Buttons …

It still comes as a constant surprise to most guys, but intercourse isn't the best way for them to push you over the edge. Here's how to get him to trigger your orgasm switch.

HIT THE C NOTE

The clitoris is your hot button to bliss! Sex researcher Shere Hite found that over 75 per cent of women need to have this little bit of flesh stimulated in order to orgasm during sex.

- ♥ Doggie-style sex leaves his hands free to go walkies all over your breasts and clitoris.
- ♥ Twirling his penis around inside your vagina will slide it against your vaginal walls while his pubic bone grinds against your clitoris. You lie face up on the floor with a couple of pillows propping up your behind. Keep your knees half-bent, your legs splayed and your arms high above your head. Your partner enters you from a high angle, planting his hands on the floor beside your head. He moves around inside you in slow figure-of-eight motions. ✪ ✪ ★★★
- ♥ Putting your feet on his buttocks when you're in missionary mode will graze his pubic bone against your clitoris. Double your pleasure by raising your legs – the higher you lift them, the deeper the penetration against the front wall of your vagina, which is where your G-spot is.
- ♥ Spreading a little water-based KY Jelly on his penis, climbing on top of him (but without putting him inside you) and then moving back and forth will put enticing pressure on your clitoris.

- ♥ Lying on your back with your legs shut adds stimulation to your clitoris, and allows more friction with the nerve-rich surface of your vagina (not to mention his penis).
- ♥ To hit your clitoris every time – MEOW! – try the coital alignment technique (also known as the CAT). Instead of entering you straight on in the missionary position, he rides high so that his pubic bone – the hard surface just above the shaft of his penis – applies pressure to the rounded bit above your vagina (the hood) where the clitoris hides. Settling into a gentle mutual rhythm in which he rocks his pubic bone back and forth over your clitoris, rather than focusing so much on thrusting in and out, you get stimulated in all the right places. ✪ ✪ ✪ ★★★

G IS FOR GLORIOUS-ASM!

Researcher Beverly Whipple discovered that halfway up the front wall of your vagina is a soft swelling that will make you scream with joy whenever it's pressed. These positions hit the G-spot's bull's-eye every time:

- ♥ Sitting on top of him, facing his feet.
- ♥ Get on top and lean backwards and forwards.
- ♥ You lie on your stomach while he gently lies on top of you so he can penetrate you deeply from behind. You'll get G-spot and clitoral sparks at the same time!
- ♥ Get underneath him and have him place his hands beneath your hips and lift your whole pelvic area into the air.

GO TO YOUR AFE ZONE

The anterior fornix erogenous is located on the front wall of the vagina, a third of the way down from the cervix. Studies have found that 95 per cent of women had not only the most orgasms, but also the most intense ones when this area was caressed.

- ♥ Rear entry is the best move for hitting your Aaah … zone.
- ♥ Slipping a pillow underneath your hips when you're on the bottom tilts your pelvis forward and has the same effect.
- ♥ Lie on your back at the end of the bed and have him stand between your legs.
- ♥ Get into the missionary position and hook your ankles around his neck.
- ♥ When your AFE area is hit, this can result in waves of muscular contractions that seem hellbent on pushing your lover right out of you. When this happens, get him to push back. The more he pushes into you forcefully, the more intense your pleasure will be.

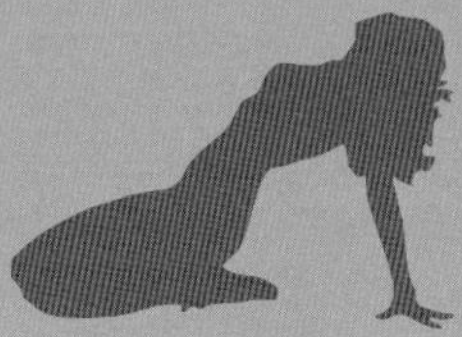

Penis Ticklers

These moves will make sure you give his favourite organ a total va-va-voom buzz during sex.

★ Whenever you're on top of him, facing his feet, consider this little trick: just as he's about to have his orgasm, grasp his toes and pull gently. It seems that the nerves in his toes are connected to the ones in his genitals so this extra stimulation increases the intensity of his ejaculation.

★ While on top, keep his penile skin stretched tight by holding it down at the base with your fingers. Imagine the heightened sensitivity you would experience if he stretched the skin around your exposed clitoris while thrusting against it with his pelvis and you'll understand why this manoeuvre can send him skyward!

★ When he's lying on top of you during sex, get him to spread his legs to take the pressure away from his testicles. If too compressed, they may become understimulated.

★ Lie flat on top of him with your legs in between his and squeeze your thighs tightly together. This way, you get to control how deeply he penetrates you while tantalizing the packed-with-nerve-endings head of his penis.

★ Double his pleasure by turning on his G-spot. When you're on top or underneath, reach behind and press on the area between his backside and balls with your forefinger.

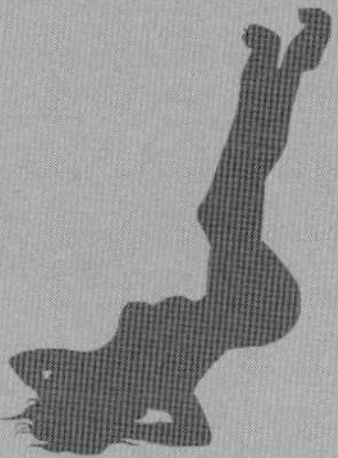

★ His penis is never happier than when it's sliding inside you as deeply as he possibly can. To give him the ground zero penetration, get into the missionary position (see page 62) and lift your legs up and apart. The higher you can go, the further he'll be able to thrust – especially if you push into him with each stroke. (It helps if you wrap your legs around his shoulders.)

★ Sit up straight on top of him – you can face either way to do this. Now grind your pelvis around and around, back and forth. At the same time, squeeze your vaginal muscles tight until you vibrate him into sex heaven.

Get Synchronized!

For a move even yummier than a five-star French meal, master the *soixante-neuf*.

★ Ask him to hum while he's giving you oral pleasure with his tongue on your pleasure knob.

★ Do the 60-minute lick. Ask for one slow, long, wet lick around your clitoris and return the favour on his love stick.

★ To prevent yourself from gagging while pleasuring him, hold the base of his penis as you suck. You'll control how deeply his penis thrusts into your mouth.

★ Up his pleasure! Play with his nipples or massage his buttocks.

Be a Movie Star

Heat up the action in your bedroom by re-enacting these steamy love scenes.

NINE AND A HALF WEEKS

Fill your fridge with lots of sticky, squishy and yummy foods like strawberries, grapes, ice cream, chocolate mousse and orange juice. Take it in turns to blindfold each other and feed and drip the food over every orifice.
✪ ★★

OUT OF SIGHT

Substitute the car boot (trunk) for any cramped, dark space (a closet will do). Slip into a short, business-like dress, then jam your bodies together on the floor in a spoon position (see page 63). He starts off by languidly stroking your thigh before roaming over the rest of your body. ✪ ✪ ★

THE POSTMAN ALWAYS RINGS TWICE

Sweep away everything from the kitchen table. Lie down on your back at the edge, extend your legs straight up, keeping them close together, and put your hands underneath your buttocks to elevate your pelvis. Standing up and gripping your legs for leverage and stability, your partner then enters you. ✪ ✪ ★★

Stretch it Out!

The looser and more supple your muscles, the more moves you can make. These stretches will help limber you into a sex gymnast!

POWER SQUATS

For overall improved hip strength and flexibility, stand with your feet slightly more than shoulder width apart and your arms straight out in front of you for balance. Bring your hips and backside back, bend your knees forward (no farther than your toes) and then straighten your legs. Do three sets of 15 repetitions a week.

BODY DIPS

Strengthen your triceps so that you can hold yourself up for longer periods when you're on top. Sit on a sturdy chair with its back securely against a wall. Hold the front of the seat on each side of your legs with the heels of your hands. Slide gently off the chair and pose, knees bent, with your elbows pointing towards the wall and your arms supporting your body. Lower your body, bending your elbows to a 90-degree angle and then push up. Do three sets of 15 repetitions a week.

HIP STRETCH

This exercise improves your range of motion when you're underneath. Lie on your back with your knees bent and your feet on the floor. Place your left foot comfortably across the middle of your right thigh, with your left thigh resting open. (For a better stretch, position your left foot closer to your hip.) Now pull your right thigh towards your chest for 20–30 seconds. Alternate sides for a total of three repetitions per side each week.

INNER THIGH AND HAMSTRING STRETCH

Limber yourself up for more athletic sexual positions. Sit down on the floor with your legs pointing outwards in a 'V' position. For a wider stretch, place your hands behind you to support yourself and push your backside forwards. Now lift it off the floor with small pelvic thrusts, then turn your upper body towards one foot. Keeping your back as flat as possible, reach for that foot with your hands. Alternate sides for a total of three reps per side every day.

PC PUMPER

Strengthening your pubococcygeus (PC) muscles enhances sexual pleasure. Do this exercise regularly and you'll be able to milk his milk his member to ecstasy while boosting your own orgasmic potential. Squeeze the muscles that control your urine flow for five seconds and then release. Do a minimum of 30 reps each day.

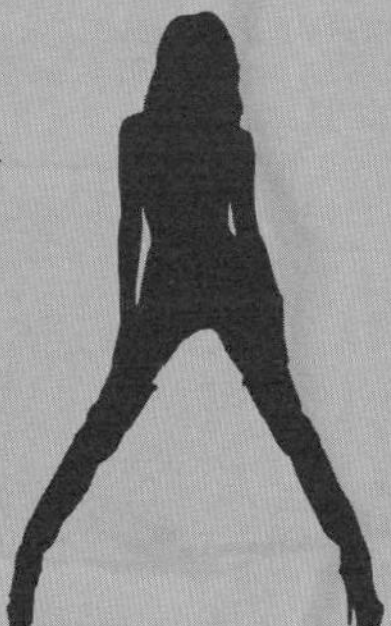

Sensual Sex

This is lovemaking that encompasses everything around you, so you slowly and steadily stimulate each other to intense peaks of sexual pleasure.

Bedroom Sexessories

Set the stage for your love ride …

★ Before making love, place mirrors all around your room so you can see your reflections from all angles. Stand up so you can press your body up against your reflection and get the erotic boost of seemingly making love to yourself.

★ Slip onto a luxurious fur throw or thick, soft rug to make love. The material feels very sensual to naked bodies.

★ All fabrics in the bedroom should be invitingly tactile – soft cotton, smooth silk, rich velvet, cool satin and knobbly bedspreads (for delicious friction).

★ Lightly scent the room or the sheets with a musky or flowery perfume. Everything else will smell fresh and clean. Eventually he'll begin to associate this scent with your lovemaking and you'll get him in the mood with just one whiff.

Use All Your Senses

When you make love, indulge in a sensual feast.

★ Create the sounds of seduction. Have him get on top. Relax your vaginal muscles as he moves up and tighten them on the downswing. With practice, you'll make a loud, sexy, squishy sound. After orgasm, ask him to stretch out so he's lying flat on top of your body. The sound of his heartbeat will reverberate through your body.

★ Give the look of love. Sitting straight up on top of him gives you a sizzling full-eye view of each other.

★ Give off sexy scents. Slip into the missionary position and lift your arms over your head to open your armpits (a sexy source of pheromones). One whiff will plunge you both into accelerated lust.

★ Indulge in a tasty turn-on. Lie on top of him so that your face is by his feet and your feet are by his head. Called a '20', this position lets you nibble each other's toes at the same time.

★ Discover the power of touch. Try making love in the dark. You have to feel your way, and not knowing where you'll be touched next can heighten the sexual tension. There's also something about being unable to see that makes your other senses respond more intensely to every sensation.

Slow-Him-Down Sex

Strike a pose and increase his staying power.

★ Change your position a few times during lovemaking. The momentary lapse can halt his momentum, which should curb early ejaculation.

★ Try the Stop/Start Technique. It doesn't matter what position you're in, but you should do most of the moving. With him lying as still as possible, gently move up and down until he nears his big moment. Stop if he's about to take an express trip to bliss until he's got himself in hand. But remember, thinking about something boring to delay ejaculation rarely works. Besides, it makes your love play slightly schizophrenic – you're turned on while he's obsessing about whether he can afford a new car! So, while all this stopping and starting is going on, he should be selfishly, happily and contentedly concentrating completely on his arousal. Once he can last as long as he wants to, he can start moving his hips as well.

★ Climbing on top and facing him gives you total control over his – and your – sensations, especially if you ride your partner while kneeling or sitting. By keeping penetration shallow, you'll be able to set the pace as slow as you want without him jumping his orgasmic gun.

★ So long as he's at least as tall as you, you can have sex in a kneeling position, even if he isn't fully erect. He sits on the raised heels of his feet and you squat over him, face to face, with your thighs spread out. Now guide his penis inside you. Once he's in, you can take some of the weight off his back by leaning back on one arm while holding onto him with the other. ✪ ✪ ★

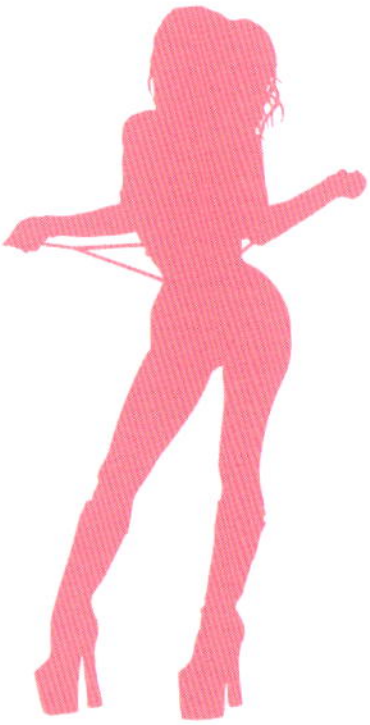

Slow Comfortable Screws

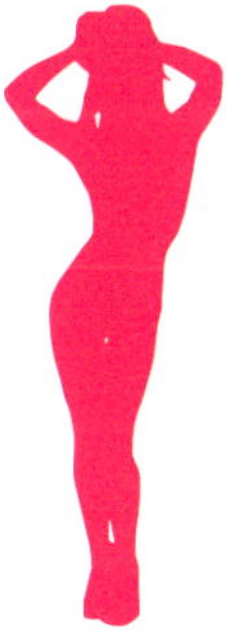

Well, you want this exquisite agony to go on for at least a few more hours, don't you?

★ To slow things down a bit, get on top or underneath. Completely relax your vaginal muscles and place your legs flat alongside his. This makes for shallower thrusts, but keep your hips rocking so your bodies know you're still interested.

★ Sit on your partner's lap with him inside you and distract each other. Lean out of the window and look at the garden, watch TV, talk about your day ... The longer you can manage to ride it out, the better the end results.

★ Moving in slow motion makes you acutely aware of every part of the movement, from the muscles and body parts you're using to your weight shifts and your breathing – all of which you miss when you move too fast. Slip into a relaxing, sensual move such as the sidestroke, with both of you lying on your sides and him curled up behind you. Tell him to insert his penis slowly while you both focus on the feeling of your skin making contact, on your breathing and on the pleasurable pressure of his penis as it advances, little by little. Take a full minute to perform what you would usually do in just one or two seconds. You'll need to towel off after this one! ✪ ★★★

★ Get into woman-on-top mode, straddling his hips. Lower yourself onto his penis, but go no farther than the glans (the very tip of it). Then lift yourself back up in retreat and repeat nine times. On the tenth repetition, lower yourself all the way down onto his penis, letting him thrust fully into your vaginal canal. Pull yourself back up and begin your next set of attack and retreat, but this time allow eight shallow thrusts and two deep ones, followed by seven shallow and three deep thrusts, and so on. By the time you're taking ten deep thrusts from him, you'll have lost count. (If you don't have strong, steely thigh muscles, try leaning forward over your partner and use your abdominal muscles to lift your pelvis up and down until you collapse in delight.)

Mood Busters

Libido lift-offs, whatever your state of mind.

WHEN YOU'RE NEW LOVERS

For first-time sex – or first-time-together sex – any position where he's on top will be the most comfortable and require the least amount of effort from you (you have enough to think about). Ease things along by placing a pillow under your hips. Another tip you might try is to push your pelvis down as he enters you to help relax things down there.

WHEN YOU HAVE YOUR PERIOD

Assume the spoon (see page 63). Then lift your top leg while he shifts his lower body into a half-kneeling position and enters you from behind. This half-doggie, half-spooning hybrid combines the cosy intimacy of lying side by side with G-spot-rubbing rear entry without ever making an issue of your period bloat. ✪ ✪ ★★★

WHEN YOU HAVE A HANGOVER

Getting the blood to rush straight to your head helps ease all that pounding, as will having a brain-melting orgasm. Studies show that an orgasm is the best cure for a headache. Start with your partner lying on his back. Facing his feet, straddle his hips on your knees and lower yourself onto his penis. Slowly extend your legs back towards his shoulders and relax your torso onto the bed or ground between his feet. Both sets of legs should now form an 'X' shape. Use your PC muscles (see page 69) and move your buttocks up and down or back and forth to maintain his erection. ✪ ✪ ★

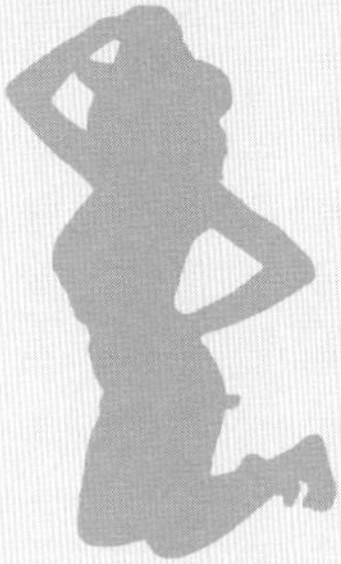

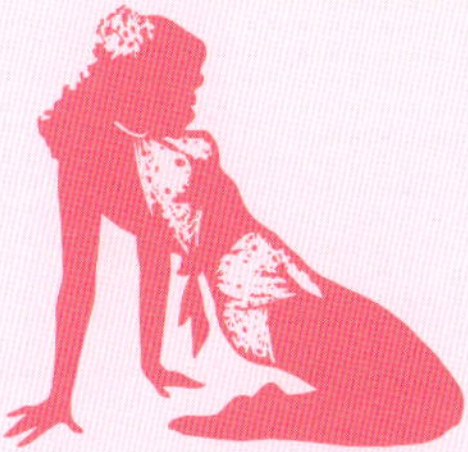

WHEN YOU'VE HAD AN ACNE ATTACK OR EATEN GARLIC FOR LUNCH

Head over heels is a sexy position that's not face to face. Kneel down, cross your arms in front of you and lean forward so that your forearms rest on the ground and your derrière is in the air (cushion your arms on a pillow if you wish). Then rest your head on your arms. Your partner stands behind you and lifts your legs up by your knees until you're almost completely vertical, then he enters you from behind. ✪ ✪ ✪ ★★

WHEN YOU HAVE PREMENSTRUAL SYNDROME

Studies have discovered two things: (1) boosted hormone levels means that right before your period is a high-octane time for you to make whoopee; and (2) an orgasm is a great cure for cramp. So, assume the position. Ask your lover to lie on his back on the bed and slowly squat onto his erect penis, facing his feet. Lean back as far as you can, being careful not to strain your lower back, and snuggle up against his chest. Reach back with your hands and caress his head. Your (bloated) tummy will look amazingly thin.
✪ ✪ ✪ ★★

WHEN YOU'RE FEELING FAT

Try a classic pose to make you look (and feel) sexy and voluptuous. Make love in a side-to-side position, propped up on your elbow with the knee of your top leg resting on the bed. To your lover, your waist will look tiny and your hips will seem ultra-curvy.

WHEN YOU'RE IN A SINGLE BED

Start in the missionary position and, with your legs and arms wrapped around him, gently roll over to one side. If there's too much weight on your bottom leg, you can carefully slip your legs between his.

Intimate Sex

Even the most vertically-challenged relationship can get stuck in the middle of orgasmic nowhere after a while. Not to worry. All you need to get your return ticket to Ecstasy-ville are a few smooth moves. Slip any of the following into your next lovefest and let the pleasure ride begin!

Spice it Up

To get things sizzling again, here are some new positions for old lovers.

THE TWISTER

Your partner lies on his back with his legs spread slightly and his head propped up with a pillow. Start by lying on your back next to him, then swing your legs over his body crosswise and keep them close together so your legs are positioned perpendicular to his. Sit on his lap and lean back on your arms for support. Open your legs slightly as he enters you and begin making slow, swivelling, corkscrew motions. ✪ ★★★

THE LEG LIFT

Your guy sits on the floor, his palms on the ground behind him and his fingers pointing away from him. His legs are splayed open and his knees are slightly bent. Placing your hands on the floor for support, you face him and straddle his lap. Raise your legs so your right leg rests on his left shoulder and your left leg is on his right shoulder. Keep your bodies close together so he doesn't slip out. The angle of his dangle will bring on deep G-spot orgasms. ✪ ✪ ✪ ★★★

THE BONDER

You and your guy lie on your sides, facing each other. Now lean in and scissor your legs together. While thrusting, hold on close to each other for leverage and to create super-close friction. Rather than typical in-and-out thrusting, this sexual scissoring lets you and your guy please each other with grinding, circular motions. ✪ ✪ ★★★

Body Boogie

Physically, not all lovers are perfect matches. Here's how to mesh your bodies in the throes of love.

WHEN YOU'RE TALLER THAN HIM

He sits on the floor with his arms stretched out behind him for support and his legs crossed loosely. You climb onto his lap so you're straddling him in a kneeling position. Hold onto his shoulders as you lower yourself onto his erect penis, Keep your bodies extremely close together as you take control of the timing and speed of the thrusting. ✪ ★★

WHEN HE'S A LOT TALLER THAN YOU

Sitting on top of him ensures your love organs stay connected.

WHEN HE HAS A LAGER GUT OR YOU'RE HEAVIER THAN HIM

A side move will let you work around your bulges. Lie on your back with your man to your right. He lies on his left-hand side. Bend and lift your right leg up. Your man arranges his right leg over your left and inserting his penis in this position allows a nice leisurely pace. Crank up the pleasure factor by grinding your buttocks tantalizingly against his pelvis. ✪✪ ★

WHEN HE PACKS A BIG ONE!

If your man has a large penis, lying flat on top of him with your legs in between his and squeezing your thighs tightly together lets you control how deeply he penetrates you, while making sure his penis still gets fully massaged. ✪ ★★★

WHEN HIS PENIS IS PUNY

The size of a penis has very little to do with satisfying a woman. All it takes is 4–5 centimetres (1½–2 inches) to reach the super-sensitive nerve endings in your vagina. And nearly every penis, no mater how tiny when flaccid, is between 12.5 and 17.5 centimetres (5 and 7 inches) when erect. But you can still make it easier for him – and for you – by opting for a rear-entry position, which will make the most of what he has. Being on top will also 'shorten' your vagina.

Putting in the Paces

According to studies, it's not the size of his package that counts – it's what you both do with it once it's in you that's the real key to how loud you'll be screaming with joy …

★ Allow him to penetrate you more deeply. Place pillows under your hips so your entire body is on an incline with your crotch angled up in the air.

★ When you're underneath, clench your buttocks. You'll lift your pelvis a little way off the bed and increase the blood flow to your pelvic area, making orgasm easier.

★ More thrusting does not necessarily mean more fun! Instead, get your man to rock your world by rocking back and forth.

★ The most sensitive nerve endings are near the opening of the vagina and in the head of the penis. So bring on a Big O by keeping penetration shallow.

★ After you've come and your vagina has tightened but your contractions are still going, ask him to keep on stroking inside your vagina until they stop. He should then quickly move to your clitoris and massage it. On the point of no return, ask him to put his fingers inside you again. Get ready to dissolve with pleasure!

★ To give him a rest while keeping him hot, ask him to stop while you do the thrusting.

Orgasms in 0 to Sexty

Here are some hurrying-up helpers for when you're having sex against the clock!

★ Do it in the morning! You're already horizontal, you have less clothes on to worry about, his testosterone level is highest, and you'll be in a carefree, glowing mood for the rest of the day.

★ Dress for speed: wear easy-to-unzip trousers (him) and a skirt with no underwear and definitely no tights (you).

★ When giving each other some simultaneous mouth sex, keep pace together by putting on some music with a strong, steady beat (pretty much anything from the 1970s will do).

★ Rear entry is best from a standing position if space is tight, but it can be tricky to match up your love organs if you and your man are different heights. For guaranteed satisfaction, face away from him and bend over so that your hands are flat on the floor and your weight is forward (or just lean against a wall).

Daring Sex

Push your acts of amour to the utmost limit. Buckle up and get ready for an action-packed ride! Here, anything goes … but proceed at your own risk – you could find yourself in a whole new position, like court!

Marathon Moments

Try some of the following moves to make your carnal connection last from here to eternity …

★ Use a water-based lubricant like KY Jelly to increase the length of time you're able to have sex without risk of soreness.

★ Leaning away from each other is the perfect beginning for a lovemaking epic, although it probably won't give either of you a pulse-pumping orgasm. Start off by sitting on top of your man, facing him. Both of you then fall back in opposite directions supporting your weight on your elbows or hands, or you can lie flat on your back (whatever makes you happy). He gently thrusts from below for as long as your hearts desire (or his penis holds out), whichever comes first! ✪ ✪ ★

★ Do the chain. Lie back with your legs up, open and wide apart while your lover lowers himself on you face down, with his head by your feet and his legs over your hips so that his feet are on either side of your shoulders. You can rest your legs on his back and play with his balls as he thrusts backwards. For a real joygasmic thrill, hold on to his hips and pull yourself up in the middle of your love play to give your insides – and his penis – a total massage. ✪ ✪ ✪ ★★★

Stay in Control

Make your contraception work for you and enjoy the double thrill of being sassy and sexy. Condoms are your best protection from AIDS, chlamydia and most other sexually transmitted diseases (STDs).

THE PILL

By suppressing ovulation, the Pill can lower your levels of testosterone. As a result, some women may feel a dip in desire. Any rear entry position gives him access to play with your clitoris as he thrusts to re-rev your cravings.

INTRAUTERINE DEVICE (IUD)

The IUD can sometimes make sex a bit dry, which can be uncomfortable. Keep things sweet and sexy by using a side-entry position where your legs are interlocked. (He has one leg on the bottom, your lower leg comes next, then his top leg, then yours).

DIAPHRAGM

Depending on the fit, this barrier device may hinder access to the area that requires stimulation. Sitting on top and leaning back so that your ankles rest on his shoulders will fully open your vagina and make sure his penis doesn't miss this hot spot during intercourse.

CERVICAL CAP

This device gives him free access to your vagina, so make good use of it! Have him come at you from behind, then rotate your hips in small, circular movements to ensure his penis bumps every part of your vaginal canal.

MALE CONDOM

Some men report reduced sensations from condoms, so up his pleasure by sitting on top of him and leaning back and forth during sex to massage his penis with your vagina.

FEMALE CONDOM

Some women find that the ring on the base stimulates their clitoris during sex. Make sure by using a man-on-top position with him riding slightly high on you.

Get Out of Bed!

Incredibly erotic hot spots for love trysts around the house will make you leap out of bed.

SOFA STRADDLER

Your partner sits back on a sofa (or comfy chair) as you straddle his lap with your legs splayed apart and your knees bent up against his chest. Then lean back so that you're almost upside-down, with your arms stretched behind you all the way to the floor to support your weight. Thrust back and forth, opening and closing your legs and clamping your PC muscles (see page 69) around him. When you're ready for him to hit his passion peak, send him soaring by squeezing your PC muscles when he's completely inside you. ✪ ✪ ✪ ★★

STAIR STOPPER

Kneel in front of your partner on the landing of a staircase, with both of you facing the stairs. While you reach up and hold onto each side of the staircase for support (or to the stairs themselves), he holds your hips and penetrates you from behind. Be careful not to pull the banisters away! ✪ ★★

TABLE ROCKER

You sit on a dresser or table and he stands, facing you. Now edge yourself down until he can comfortably slip inside you. This body-rocking move angles your vagina just right for a two-for-one G-spot/clit climax. ✪ ✪ ★★★

WATER PLAY

He gets in the bath first with his back to one end, his legs spread out in front of him and his knees slightly bent. (If your bath has taps at one end, make sure this is the way his back is facing.) Now you get in, sitting so you're facing him, with your arms propping you up from behind. Position your legs so they're bent on either side of him and your feet are resting lightly against the edge of the bath (if the bath isn't big enough to get a stable surface, just wrap your legs around his waist). Push your pelvis forward, lift your hips a little and use one hand to put him inside you. ✪ ✪ ✪ ★

ON THE WASHING MACHINE

Have him sit on the washing machine. Then climb onto his lap, facing away from him (he can keep you in place by encircling you in his arms). Flip on the spin cycle and get ready to vibrate yourselves to a deliciously dirty climax. ✪ ✪ ★★★

The Great Outdoors

Whatever the scenery, the lack of a ceiling (and the risk of being spotted) will intensify the experience outside. If you're going to have sex outdoors in any position other than standing, bring a soft blanket with you.

ON THE BEACH

Making love on the beach can be a truly sexy. Use the rhythm of the waves to roll from underneath to on top and back again – you'll come oceans!

ON A PARK BENCH

Wear a long, floaty skirt without underwear and have him wear easy-access shorts. Keep things discreet by lifting your skirt, sitting on his lap side-saddle and wriggling gently until you achieve the desired effect.

ON THE GRASS

Relax on your stomach and elbows, and get your man to lie on top of you with his weight on his arms. Raise your hips slightly to increase penetration.

ON A CAR BONNET

Make sure the engine is cool and the car alarm is switched off! Then lie back with your hips at the edge of the bonnet (hood) and your legs spread wide. He stands between your legs, lifts them and penetrates you. Pull up to the bumper, baby!

IN A PARK

Stand facing a wall or tree with your feet about 45 centimetres (18 inches) apart. He stands behind you, bends his knees and enters you from below. If he wants to show off, he can hold your hips and lean back, while you lean forward against the wall.

Go Wild

Rev up the raunch with some lurve tools and keep things sweet between the sheets.

★ There's nothing like feathers to tickle his fancy. Have a wide assortment handy – a feather duster, a boa, a quill, a peacock feather. Lightly brush over his whole love organ area while you sit on top of him.

★ Give him a lap dance. Dress in crotchless panties and have your partner lean back on a strong, comfortable chair. Facing him and with your hands behind you resting on his knees, snuggle onto his lap. Lift your ankles up to rest on his shoulders. Start gyrating by inching yourself back and forth against his erect member. Slip him in and out of you to drive him wild with desire.

★ Put a small scoop of your favourite ice scream in your vagina, lie back and slip him inside you. Alternate with dripping warm – but not hot – wax over your bodies (be very careful, you don't want to cause third-degree burns!) to make your blood vessels dance with delight and give him a temperature-raising orgasm. Or try something bubbly like soda or champagne.

★ Have him tie your hands and feet together, then set you up on your elbows and knees. He then comes from behind to ravish you mercilessly.

★ If you have long hair, climb on top of him so you can seductively brush it back and forth across his body during sex.

★ Get fruity! A mashed banana or peaches inserted in your vagina is a delightful invitation for him to whoosh his penis around in it. Once you climax, switch to the 69 position for sweet afters.

★ Cool down your vagina with a flavoured ice-cream stick, then replace it with his penis. The heat of his organ against your icy skin will create a sizzling sensation.

★ Wrap a silk scarf around your hand to stroke him. Rub it all over his body, tying it around his penis or testicles. Then use it to tie his hands or feet together and climb on top of him.

★ Get on the fast track to ecstasy! Lie back in the missionary position and have him slip a vibrator against the base of your clitoris while he's inside you. He'll be able to feel the vibrations too and soon you'll both be pulsating with pleasure.

Join the Club

To become a member, the only requirement is body-blistering sex!

THE MILE-UNDER CLUB

Go scuba diving in warm water so you can wear just a bathing suit (this move also works well in waist-high water). Push the crotch of your bathing suit aside, then wrap your legs tightly around his waist (the water will make you lighter than air). Go with the flow, using the motion of the water to rock you up and down.

THE FAST-LANE CLUB

If you get the hots while driving your car, pull over in a secluded spot and jump on his lap. You can either face him with your knees pushed against your chest and your feet on the seat or hooked over the neck rest, or face away from him with your feet on the car floor. Either way, you won't be able to get much movement, so squeeze your thighs to increase the pressure on your love organs.

THE FAR-OUT CLUB

Doing it in a boat is like making love on a waterbed! But the position you choose isn't as important as how you position yourselves in the boat. Stand close to the centre of the boat and keep your body low. Motor boats and catamarans are the most stable, canoes the least. (Whatever you do, don't remove personal flotation devices and make sure you can both swim!)

Spiritual Sex

Your guide to nookie nirvana. Get ready to have the best, most satisfying, intense, mind-blowing sexual experience of your life. But be warned – there's no such thing as a spiritual quickie. Love made Eastern-style can last for hours (read: hours of pure soul-in-sync bliss ... mmmm!).

Say Ohm-My-God!

Prime your body for divine passion.

THE BRIDGE

Sit face to face with your legs wrapped around each other's backs. Slip him inside you and snuggle in by grasping each other's elbows, then lean back. Now see if you can tilt your head far enough back to rest it on the floor. Try to remain still and concentrate on your bodies, completely connecting the sexual energies flowing through you. ✪ ✪ ★★

THE JUMPING FROG

Start in the standard missionary position. He then rises up on all fours, and you raise your pelvis to meet his penis. As he stays stationary, start moving your hips up and down to get him jumping. ✪ ✪ ★★

THE CRANE

Stand facing your partner with your left foot turned out, perpendicular to your sweetheart, and your right foot forward. His legs should be slightly bent, spaced about 1 metre (3 feet) apart. With your arms resting on his shoulders and his arms around your lower back, slowly pull your right leg up and prop your right foot on his shoulder. Once he penetrates you, ease into the vertical split by sliding your right calf as far up his shoulder as you comfortably can. ✪ ✪ ★★

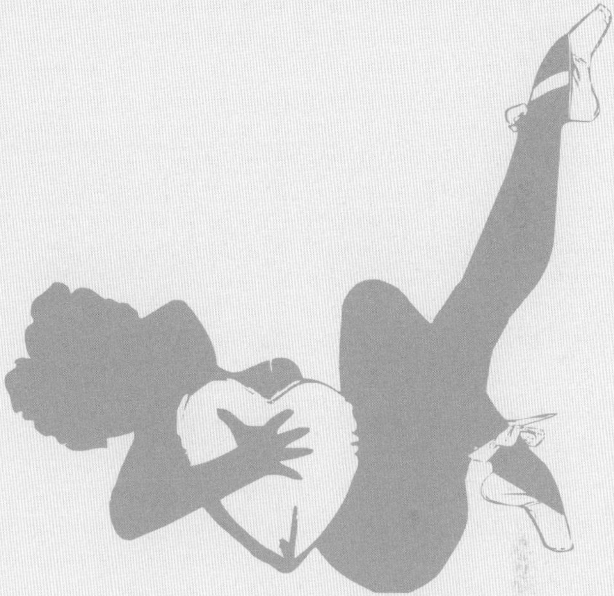

THE THREE-POINTED STAR

Lie on your back with your left leg extended straight up in the air and your right leg stretched out to your right on the floor, perpendicular to your body. Reach out across the floor with your right hand and clasp your right knee, forming a triangle with your right side, right leg and right arm. Your partner crouches at the bottom and enters you.

✪ ★★★

Read Your Horoscope

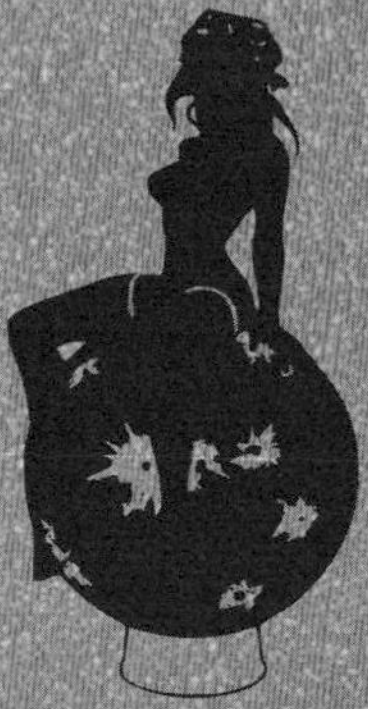

Follow your zodiac to discover the most out-of-this-world position for you …

ARIES

An ultra-physical lover who like to take charge of her own sexuality.
BEST MOVE: Anything on top that lets you masturbate yourself to orgasm while controlling the thrusting.

TAURUS

A sensual lover who likes sex to last.
BEST MOVE: A side-by-side position that lets you do it just how you like it: in long, lazy bouts, with plenty of time out for kissing and caressing.

GEMINI

She likes variety, and lots of it!
BEST MOVE: Start on top, so you're sitting straight up facing your lover. You can then lean forwards and backwards, or even swivel around to face his feet or roll over so you're underneath.

CANCER

A shy lover – she's never the aggressor.
BEST MOVE: The classic missionary position lets you feel like you're being seduced, especially if he holds your hands tight above your head.

LEO

She loves the foreplay almost more than she enjoys the intercourse.
BEST MOVE: Doing the 69 really lets you indulge your oral side.

VIRGO

Sexually mercurial, the Virgo lover likes to try many different things.
BEST MOVE: Just about anything will spark your interest – and orgasms!

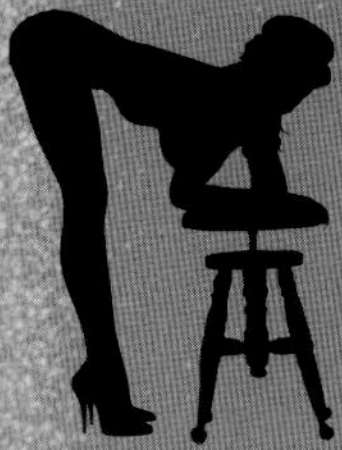

LIBRA

For her, it's all about the pursuit of pleasure ...

BEST MOVE: Rear entry, so you or your lover can caress your clitoris at the same time.

SCORPIO

Lusty and passionate, she likes to direct the action.

BEST MOVE: Anything that puts you on top and in control of the depth and pace.

SAGITTARIUS

A strong lover, she enjoys strenuous intercourse and will make love through the night.

BEST MOVE: Sitting on top and leaning back so you can see your lover as he massages your clitoris and breasts.

CAPRICORN

A straightforward and direct lover, she doesn't relish complicated sex.

BEST MOVE: The straightforward man-on-top move keeps things simple and sexy.

AQUARIUS

Curious and uninhibited, the Aquarian likes to make love whenever – and wherever – the urge strikes.

BEST MOVE: Usually standing and leaning over for a sexy quickie.

PISCES

An unusually creative lover who believes in the possibility of total ecstasy.

BEST MOVE: You take classic poses just that little bit further. Lifting your legs over his shoulders while sitting on top of him, or sitting on his lap with your legs intertwined are two ways you might put your own stamp on making love.

Chapter 4
Orgasms

Oooohh!
Orgasm Training Tips

According to sex pros Masters and Johnson, 10 per cent of women have never experienced the melting sensation of the Big O. But that doesn't mean they're ice queens. After all, orgasms aren't a basic instinct; they're a learned technique. Here are some sexercises that'll make you moan with delight:

★ Masturbation is the surest path to orgasm for both sexes – most people can bring themselves to ecstasy in four minutes flat. And research shows that the more orgasms you have by any means, the more orgasms you will have overall. Women who regularly let their fingers do the walking require less time to become aroused, have significantly more orgasms, greater sexual desire, higher self-esteem and greater marital and sexual satisfaction.

★ Practise, Practise, Practise. Sex is like any other exercise. The more you do it, the better you become at it and the more you will enjoy it – the chemicals in your brain guarantee this. If you start making love more often, the chemical communication between brain cells quickens and intensifies because the impulses are travelling on a well-beaten path. The pay-off is more orgasms with less effort.

★ One fact that was probably left out of your biology class was the 'Use It' or 'Lose It' theory of sex. Sexual abstinence in women causes what's known as 'vaginal atrophy' – a general drying and closing-up of the vagina to the point where intercourse becomes virtually impossible. But studies have shown that women who stay sexually active, either with a partner or through self-stimulation, clock in more orgasms.

★ Get a massage. It increases the blood flow that warms your vaginal muscles so they'll more easily and perform to their fullest capacity.

★ Have what's known as an active orgasm. During intercourse, bear down, pushing the same muscles as though you are trying to expel something from your vagina. This helps you to push down against the penis or squeeze it up into you. The result: a longer and deeper orgasm. And it'll make his penis stand up and pay attention as well!

★ Buff pelvic floor muscles (the ones you clench when you're desperate for a pee) mean bigger, more intense and just plain more orgasms for men and women. Another benefit: the clitoris rests on these muscles, so the exercises also strengthen the clitoris and lead to stronger sensations. Start by squeezing and releasing the muscles 15 times a day, twice each day. Don't hold the contraction; just squeeze and let go. You can do the exercise anywhere: while driving a car, watching TV, during a meeting. (Just don't announce it to everybody, okay?) Gradually increase the number of squeezes until you're doing about 75, two times a day.

★ Working out for around an hour before your sex play gets you hot in every sense of the word. Any kind of vigorous physical exercise helps stimulate the blood flow and boosts aerobic conditioning, which preps the body for a meltdown orgasm. Also, studies show that people who exercise at least three times a week are more in tune with their bodies and more likely to be sexually responsive.

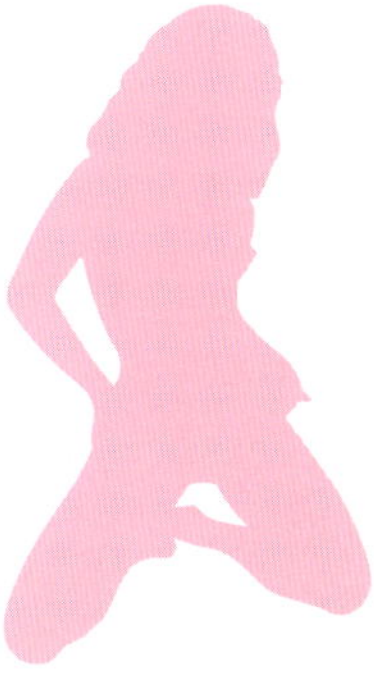

Oh!Oh!Oh!Oh! Sensory Orgasms

You have five built-in tools to help you achieve orgasm – here's how to use them:

1 **TOUCHING**
The reason why studies find that only 30 per cent of women orgasm during intercourse is because women really need stimulation to the clitoris. But this little magic button is not a minipenis. The best touch? It's one that moves around your love button rather than one that applies pressure directly onto it.

2 **SEEING**
Seeing: Use your eyes as well as your hands and mouth. Just at the moment of orgasm, look deep into each other's eyes. An Archives of Sexual Behaviour study found that the erotic image of your lover in the throes of pleasure is an incredible turn-on for both men and women. You can close your eyes and have an individual experience, but if you keep them open, it's a shared one.

3 **TASTE**
Chocolate is known to contain natural feel-good chemicals that can boost the sweetness of your orgasm. Smear each other with chocolate body paint and slowly lick it off.

4 **SMELL**
Women are more sensitive to pheromones – substances secreted by the body with an often undetectable odour that stimulates sexual desire. Nuzzling his armpit during orgasm can give you a heady whiff of his scent that'll make you swoon with bliss.

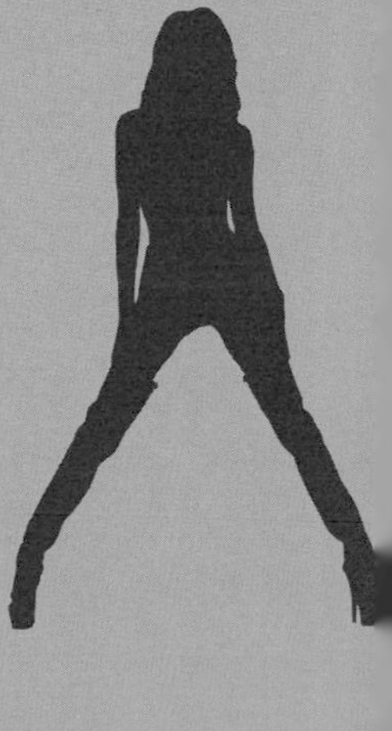

5 HEARING

If you are going through a lean period orgasm-wise or just can't seem to get yourself in the mood, you might want to try role-playing. This is not – repeat not – faking orgasm. Role-playing is when you try to cheer your orgasm into action when it seems to be hovering just around the corner. Exaggerate your movements and sounds – wriggle, clench, moan. Now throw in a few 'yes, baby, yes' screams. The whole idea here is to encourage your responsiveness and cheerlead your orgasm into action.

No-Hands Orgasms

According to sex therapists, the best sex starts in the brain...

★ Think that you are enjoying yourself and you will. According to studies by Louisiana-based sex researcher Eileen Palace, PhD, when women learn to raise their expectations about sex, their bodies become more responsive within 30 seconds.

★ In her research on easily-orgasmic women, Gina Ogden, PhD, found that 64 per cent had experienced orgasm through fantasy or dreams alone, without any touch.

★ A *Journal of Sex Research* study found 46 per cent of women and 38 per cent of men regularly indulge in erotic daydreams to keep their love juices flowing. In fact, in some cases, fantasies made all the difference between experiencing an incredible climax or none at all.

★ Often the reasons for lacklustre orgasms have little to do with our bodies. Cutting out distractions like the phone, work stress and life worries helps you relax, and that helps to speed both your own and your partner's arousal along by widening the arteries of the vagina and penis so blood flows in freely to swell the tissues.

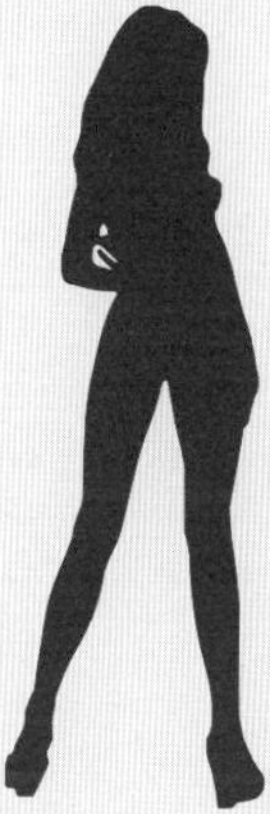

★ Of course, physical foreplay is an important part of a good sexual experience, but mental foreplay is equally significant. Planning ahead makes your body far more responsive and primes it for orgasm.

★ Concentrate on your own feelings during sex. Women are so often concerned with pleasing their partners or worried about their failure to reach orgasm that they can't fully relax and go with their own flow.

★ Have an emotional orgasm. People think of sex as a very mechanical thing: How big?, how often?, how many times did I have an orgasm?, how long did it take? When we think of sex that way, something is lost – namely, the emotional component that bonds you and your man; the key to sweeter sex. When you catch yourself calculating – what should I do?, how hard? and for how long? – refocus your thoughts and try to concentrate on how close you feel to him.

★ The ultimate no-hands experience is known as the extragenital orgasm (no vaginal contact). While 10 per cent of women have this talent naturally, anyone can develop sexy brain power – just replay your favourite erotic images in your mind (if you need inspiration, flip through a sexy magazine). Soon, you'll be able to mentally bring on the Big O wherever you are.

Pleasure Timetable

The timing of a sexual encounter – the day of the month and even the hour of the day – can have a distinct impact on the quality of your orgasms.

★ The Kinsey Institute found that only 7.7 per cent of the women whose lovers spent 21 minutes or longer on foreplay failed to reach orgasm.

★ Synchronize your pleasure by giving each other a tongue bath at the same time. Lie head-to-toe and use your mouths as you would your love organs – imitate the grip of your vagina on his penis by contracting and sucking his tool. Meanwhile, he slides a firm tongue in and out of you. Get into a rhythm and then keep it up until you're both swallowed up in mutual ecstasy.

★ Do it during your period. The high levels of progesterone in your body will give you one of the raunchiest orgasms you've ever had. (It's also good for suppressing period pains!)

★ Right before ovulation and around the time you menstruate are two tidal waves of orgasmic energy... get a surfboard and have a fun ride.

★ Turn 30. Studies from The Kinsey Institute show that compared to their twenties, when only 23 per cent of women regularly experience orgasm, by 30 around 90 per cent of them do.

★ Strange as it may sound, many people tend to have sex at precisely the wrong time, physiologically speaking – at the end of the day when they're fatigued, stiff, full from dinner and so least likely to be able to be turned on orgasmically.

★ Testosterone levels are highest when we first wake up, and they decrease as the day progresses, which means your best orgasms are most likely to happen when you make love first thing in the morning.

★ Come first. In one survey of 805 nurses, the women who reported the least trouble in reaching orgasm were those whose partners had delayed their own orgasms until the women experienced theirs. The Stop-Start technique (every time he is close to orgasm, you stop stimulating him until he can regain control) slows him down.

Don't Stop! Moregasms

Or how to have as many moments of pure bliss as you desire...

★ Women who regularly leap from one orgasm to another report varied stimulation is the key. Once you've climaxed, simply change the body part being caressed or your lovemaking position (and therefore the type and location of stimulation).

★ Keep going. The beauty of the clitoris is that it doesn't need to have any R&R (rest and relaxation) after climaxing. As long as it gets stimulation, you'll keep on coming. (One of the women who took part in a study had a staggering 134 moments of bliss in a row.)

★ A State University of New York Health Science Centre at Brooklyn study found that men can actually learn to climax and keep their erection through three to ten orgasms before exploding in the usual way. The key lies in helping him raise his orgasmic threshold by constantly approaching, then, just before he reaches the point of no return, backing away from ejaculation. Stimulate, then stop and rest; stimulate, then stop and rest. According to the study, this helps men to separate the sensation of orgasm from the experience of ejaculation. And the physical result? He'll experience all the explosive feelings of orgasm without the ejaculation as often as he desires. And the emotional result? He'll adore you forever.

★ Have a sequential orgasm. This means a series of climaxes which come close together – anywhere from one to ten minutes apart – with a slight dip in your arousal in between. Oral sex followed by intercourse is all it takes.

The One-Hour Orgasm

Five quick ways to have an endless orgasm...

1 Take a minute to do what you'd normally do in two seconds. Moving in slow motion makes you acutely aware of every sensation.

2 Leaning away from each other is perfect for beginning a lovemaking marathon. Sit on top of your man, facing him. Now both of you fall back in opposite directions with your weight on your elbows or hands, or lie flat on your back (whatever makes you happy). He can gently thrust from below for as long as your heart's desire (or his penis holds out) – whichever comes first.

3 A sex-surrogate technique called 'vaginal containment' makes his erection – and your pleasure – last forever. Straddle him or lie on top, with his penis inside you. He shouldn't move at all; he just concentrates on enjoying the sensation of containment.

4 Hit the right nerves and sexual euphoria can reach new stratospheres. Research shows that the two genital nerves that surround the pelvic floor muscles give two kinds of erotic sensation. The first is a sharp twinge that occurs when the clitoris or base of the penis is erect and caressed; the second is a warm, melting feeling that happens when the inside of the vagina or the shaft of the penis is stimulated to climatic heights. Experience both types, one after another, in a single love fest, and you'll have what's called a blended orgasm, which can last for up to an hour.

5 Recalibrate him. You can teach your man to last longer, plus give him a more explosive orgasm. While stroking his penis with your hand, ask him to rate his arousal on a scale of one to ten, with ten being orgasm. The idea here is to bring him to several peaks and then back down again without him climaxing. When he says he's reached a relatively low four, stop and tell him to breathe until his arousal subsides a hit. Now, rev him up to a heart-pounding eight, then stop until he's back down to a six or so. Finally, take him all the way.

Now! All the Right Moves...

Most women are well equipped to have an orgasm during intercourse. It's simply a matter of putting yourself in the best position to experience heaven...

★ For a truly explosive orgasm, squat on your partner (who is sitting up). Now thrust towards each other ten times. Stop and then squeeze powerfully with your pelvic floor muscles (see pages 172–3) ten times.

★ Give his and your love organs a massage in the middle of intercourse for a real orgasmic thrill. Lie back with your legs up, open and wide apart while he lowers himself on you face down, with his head by your feet and his legs over your hips so that his feet are on either side of your shoulders. Then hold onto his hips and pull yourself up a few inches. Repeat until you collapse.

★ Factor in the state of your more the weight of you and your down and make hitting the most less likely. For best results, mattress: The softer it is, the partner will push your pelvis sensitive parts of your vagina try the floor instead.

★ Studies have found that 77 per cent of women climax when they use the coital alignment technique (also known as the CAT). Your lover climbs on top, à la the Missionary, but instead of entering you straight on, he lies so his weight is totally on top of you and his pubic bone is actually rubbing against your clitoris. By settling into a gentle rocking rhythm, his penis rubs against your clitoris while moving in and out of your vagina.

Up Your Ecstasy Odds

Three simple variations will up your ecstasy odds exponentially when using the Missionary position:

1 Your lover raises his body, resting his weight on his elbows or his outstretched arms. This puts greater pressure on your clitoris.

2 He puts his legs outside yours, while you keep yours together. This will give you lots of friction.

3 Raising your legs so that your knees are pressed to your chest and your legs are draped over his shoulders will make your vagina longer, allowing him to penetrate you more deeply. This will give you more friction and pressure exactly where you crave it most of all – your vaginal lips and clitoris.

For the ultimate hot-spot position, place two stacks of firm towels together to form two sets of comfortable piles a few feet apart. Now face each other so that your backs are against the pillows. Arrange your bodies so one partner's legs are wrapped around the other's and your genitals easily connect. This position will stimulate multiple erogenous zones for both of you. You can vary the sensation if he pulls all the way out on some strokes and rubs his penis against your clitoris before thrusting in again. And the other advantage of this position? Four hands free!

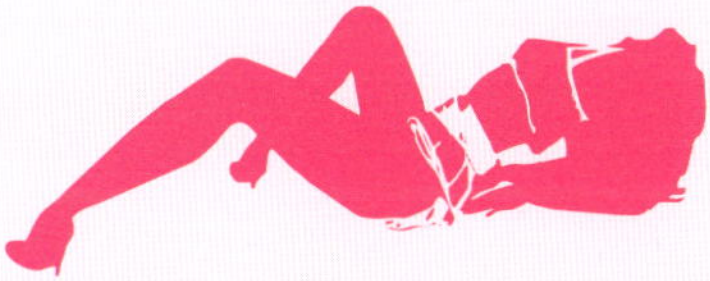

Satisfaction Guaranteed

These tips promise to please:

★ At something like 2,000 cycles per minute, the vibrator will send you both so high, you'll need clearance to land. If you don't have access to a sex shop, cheat by getting a battery-powered massager from the chemist. Don't worry about the shape – researchers have found it's the vibrations, not the shape, that triggers orgasm. Place it against your skin near the clitoris (but not directly on it, which can be too painful and intense).

★ Making love on a dryer during the spin cycle has a similar effect to using a vibrator.

★ If he tends to come before you and then immediately drops off to sleep, try the Dual-Stimulation technique. Select an intercourse position in which your partner (or you) can easily reach your clitoris (such as the rear entry). This extra bit of stimulation may be all that you need to send you straight to heaven and back.

★ Lay back and do ... nothing. NOT trying for an orgasm is the surest way to have one.

★ After you've climaxed, your vagina will tighten up and then contract. If your lover alternates stroking the inside of your vagina with your clitoris, you'll keep on feeling the contractions every five seconds or so until you're completely taken over by delicious waves of pleasure.

★ Get stressed out. Conventional wisdom says that anxiety keeps us from climaxing. Yet there is also evidence to demonstrate that anxiety can increase sexual arousal by wonderfully concentrating the mind – in the same way that pre-curtain butterflies improves an actor's performance.

★ Get out while the sun shines. Just 15 consecutive minutes of exposure to sunlight signals your brain to release the feel-good chemical serotonin, making it easier for you to orgasm when the time comes.

Take Charge of Your Pleasure

We often think of an orgasm as something which happens to us. Yet all it takes is a little know-how to control of your own pleasure...

★ You can programme yourself to have a coital orgasm (i.e., through intercourse as opposed to clitoral stimulation) using the Bridge technique. Your partner (or you) touches your clitoris while he is moving in and out of you. At the point of your climax, you stop stimulating and concentrate on the rhythm of his strokes as you orgasm. Each time you have sex, stop stimulating your clitoris a little earlier: the penetration will become the trigger for your mental Big O.

★ One technique sex therapists recommend to heighten intensity is to hover at the brink of orgasm for as long as possible. Orgasm is really just the release of extreme body tension. So the more tension you have in your body, the more pleasurable the release will be. Savour the bliss of being almost, but not quite there by backing off as you both get close to the Big O. Move to a less-sensitive area for a few minutes, then build the excitement back up again. You can increase and decrease your arousal a few times before surrendering to a head-to-toe burst of pure pleasure.

★ Clenching your buttocks and your upper thigh muscles helps increase blood flow to your entire pelvic area. This increased blood flow translates into greater vaginal lubrication and clitoral engorgement, which is believed to push the nerve receptors closer to the vaginal wall for greater sensation. Just be sure not to hold your breath as you squeeze your behind – it oxygenates the muscles, making your contractions more efficient.

★ Anything that presses down on part of your lower abdomen during intercourse (his hand, your hand or squeezing the muscles or even doing a mini sit-up) massages your inner clitoris, putting you over the orgasmic edge.

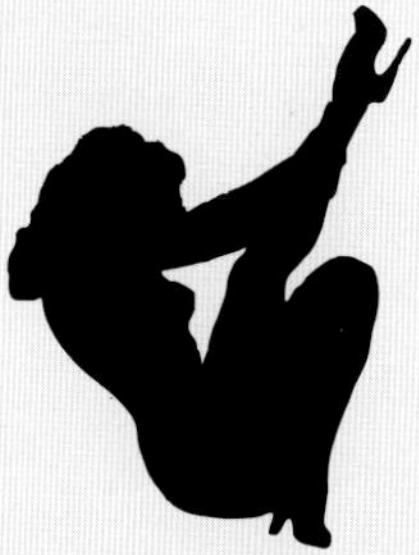

Yes!Yes!Yes!

Breathless orgasms... In the heat of passion, how you breathe is probably the last thing you probably want to be thinking about. But, surprisingly, changing your breathing pattern can help increase an orgasm's impact. The faster you breathe, the more excited you get.

★ Training the diaphragm, the muscular partition that separates the chest and abdominal cavity, can really increase the intensity of your orgasm. Practise puffing out through your mouth, huff-huff-huff-huff, concentrating on bringing each out-breath up from your belly, so you feel your diaphragm contracting to force the air out. Then during sex, as you feel an orgasm approach, try breathing more strongly and consciously than usual to force each breath out from your diaphragm. You'll increase the tension through your whole abdomen and upper body, raising the intensity of your ecstasy.

★ Position yourself so that your head is hanging off the end of the bed. This increases blood flow to your head and changes your breathing pattern, mounting the feelings of sexual tension and arousal.

★ Breathing through your nose is good for de-stressing yourself, but for truly great sex you need to breathe deeply through your mouth.

★ Deep breathing from the stomach instead of the chest during sex will relax you and increase the flow of sexual energy around your body. When you breathe in, push your stomach in as flat as it will go. As you release, push out and hold to the count of five. This makes you feel more energetic, increases your sensitivity to sex and slows down your reactions so you can really take pleasure in them.

★ Sex therapists advise women who have trouble reaching orgasm to change their breathing patterns. (If you hold your breath, exhale and vice versa.)

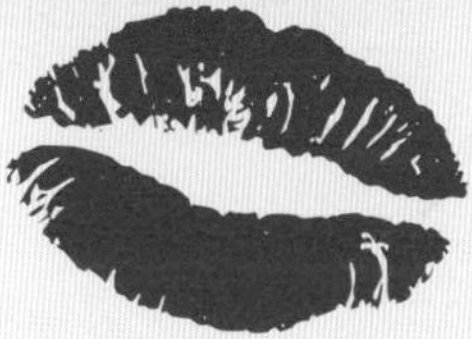

Mouthwatering Orgasms

Turn your orgasms into a delicious sexperience.

★ Try teaching him the Zen principle of oral pleasure: You can't 'see' pleasure in a woman, but you can feel it. With this in mind, he should place his tongue flat against your clitoris – the more it pulses, the hotter you are.

★ Remind him that his tongue is not a mini version of his penis. He should keep it soft and flat, and think of licking an ice-cream cone rather than plunging it in and out like a hydraulic drill.

★ The average woman needs her lover to spend about 20 minutes 'downtown' in order to make her body salsa.

★ Join your hand and mouth together to hold his penis. Move them up and down in a slow and steady rhythm. This is seriously orgasmic – it will feel like a hot vagina with magic fingers.

★ Make his entire body curl with pleasure by cradling his penis between your breasts as you lick him.

★ Most men prefer you underneath, like an oral Missionary position. One professional trick is to lie with your head thrown back over the edge of the bed to make your throat form one long, erotic passage.

★ Find a rhythm during oral sex. Being in tune with each other's body signals – following breathing patterns, body movements and hip gyrations – will all help to keep you on orgasmic track.

On-the-Spot Bliss

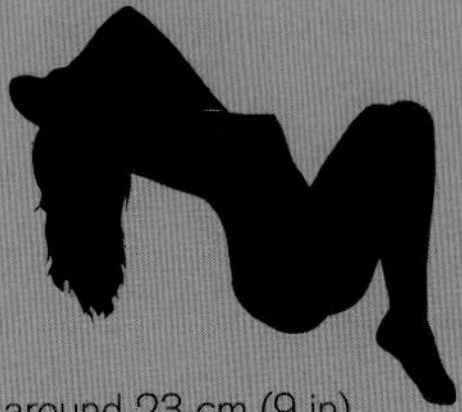

YOU

★ Rather than just a mini-knob of flesh, research published in the *Journal of Urology* confirms that the clitoris is also composed of around 23 cm (9 in) of highly sensitive erectile tissue that extends along the belly side of the vaginal wall. When stimulated in the right way, this inner clitoris can set off melt-down orgasms.
BEST MOVE: Straddle him and lean back to push his penis against the front wall of your vagina.

★ The urethra, the tiny area of tissue below the clitoris that you pee from, is actually a sexual pleasure point.
BEST MOVE: The urethra is a good place to shift his tongue or mouth after you've had an orgasm and your clitoris is feeling too sensitive for continued direct stimulation.

★ Achieve maximum pleasure by having him stimulate all three parts of what is called the orgasmic crescent – a curved area that extends from the clitoral tip across the urethral opening to the G-spot (see below).
BEST MOVE: Using tongue, hands or both, your lover should touch both the clitoral tip and the U-spot, while simultaneously pressing the G-spot.

★ The G-spot is a sensitive mass of tissue one-third of the way up the front wall of the vagina (it feels like a soft marshmallow when touched). When pressed, it sets off an orgasm that is deeper and more of a full pelvic wave compared to the quick succession of mini-explosions from a clitoral orgasm.
BEST MOVE: Kneel at the edge of the bed, with your lover standing and entering you from behind.

★ According to a study published in the *Journal of Sex Research*, the cervix and the clitoris may be part of the same nerve network, which explains why, for roughly half of all women, stimulation of the cervix can lead to an intense orgasm.
BEST MOVE: Try sitting on top of your partner while facing his feet for the deepest penetration.

HIM

★ Stroking his frenulum – the vertical ridge that extends from the tip to the shaft of the penis – will hit his climax switch. Not only are there more nerve endings there, but the skin is also extremely thin.
BEST MOVE: Clench your pelvic muscles just as he pulls out will give his F-spot a massage.

★ Many men are quite surprised to discover the range and depth of the sensation when you stroke their raphe – the visible line along the centre of the scrotum. They may even end up ejaculating sooner than they (and you) originally planned.
BEST MOVE: Excite the raphe by gently running your fingertips along it.

★ A man's erection doesn't end at the base of the penis. There's a railroad junction full of nerves in the perineum – that smooth triangle of flesh between the base of his penis and his anus which, when pressed, will send him into an orgasmic swoon.
BEST MOVE: Gently rub the spot with the pad of your finger or thumb. (Pressing really hard with one forceful push can actually stop him from peaking, so be careful.)

★ Owing to its location at the base of the penis, a man's erection is more or less anchored upon the prostrate (also known as the male G-spot).
BEST MOVE: Slip a well-lubricated finger through the rectum and probe the rounded back wall of the prostrate. When you start to feel a firm, rounded walnut-size lump, gently caress it while stroking his penis at the same time.

BOTH OF YOU...

★ The anus is an often-missed hot spot, but it is crammed with sensitive nerves guaranteed to raise the orgasmic quotient.
BEST MOVE: A well-lubricated finger gently slipped into the bottom just as climax hits.

★ Find your hidden hot spot. Make a fist and note where your middle finger hits your palm. Reflexologists believe stimulating this site, which corresponds with the heart centre, helps ignite your orgasm. Before sex, press the spot rhythmically with the thumb of your other hand for 15 seconds, then gently rotate the thumb there for 15 seconds. Repeat three times and then switch hands.

Cosmic Sex

How to achieve joygasmic nirvana:

He sits upright with his legs bent at the knees, but wide apart. You sit on top of him with your legs over his while you support his upper body. Now you both move in a rhythmic and slow fashion, while concentrating on deep breathing techniques. According to Taoists, this is the ultimate position to be in while the body orgasms.

Tantrics embrace each other's aura (energy fields said to buzz around each of us) for full-body orgasms. Start by imagining yourselves encircled in a glowing orb of light. Now, facing each other, he puts his Arrow of Love (figure it out) in your Seat of Pleasure as you lie back. Don't move: instead, just concentrate on breathing and looking into each other's eyes. Try to hold out for half an hour – the result will be heavenly.

The Kama Sutra describes over 2,000 positions – all guaranteed to make you explode. Try the Mare, one of the easier moves. He sits, legs out, and hands behind him for support. You're on top, with your back to him, kneeling on either side of his legs.

60-Second Climaxes

Follow the next few tips and you'll climax before you finish reading this sentence.

The moves that work best when you're in a hurry are generally carried out standing up, especially if space is tight. Unfortunately, the male and female physique rarely match up in a way that makes this feasible. Doing it on the stairs (with you one step higher) – or on an incline – evens things out. The same goes for bending over, with your bum towards his groin. In fact, anything done in the rear entry position gives the deep penetration often needed for quick sex and lets his penis hit the ultra-sensitive front of your vaginal wall.

Some women get an overwhelming orgasm from quick intercourse without foreplay, but with deep penetration and they say that it feels different from the orgasms they get from clitoral stimulation or less vigorous intercourse. This sort of orgasm produces gasping, breath-holding, and a once-and-for-all climax. Too much foreplay derails this special response, which – when it happens – is as rapid as any man's.

In one survey, which was conducted by Bowling Green State University, the majority of women polled reported that they preferred 'hard, driving sex' to the 'slow, gentle' kind. Researchers concluded that since the vagina is most sensitive in its outer third part, women need to have constant pressure to orgasm during sex.

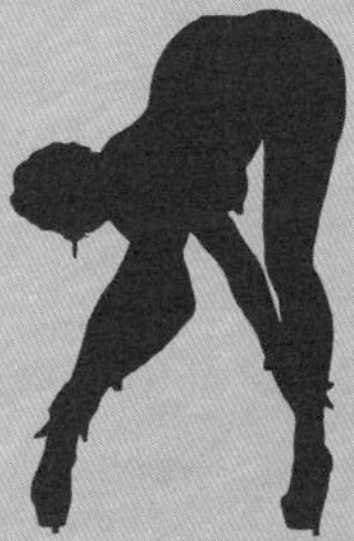

Ahhhh! Orgasm Secrets

These little-known facts about your orgasms may be just the insider knowledge you need to up your pleasure quotient...

★ Rest up. When you're exhausted, you just don't have the stamina needed to achieve powerful orgasms.

★ If you're running dry, don't assume you're not interested. You can lubricate without being aroused, and vice versa. Lubrication is influenced by numerous outside factors – your menstrual cycle, whether you drink or smoke, medications like antihistamines and/or how much stress you're experiencing. The simplest solution is to add spit to the mix – yours or his – or water. Otherwise, invest in a commercial lubricant (note for latex protection users: oil-based products destroy the latex) or condoms with extra lubrication.

★ Drink lots of water and skip the trip to the toilet before sex. Sex researcher Estelle Lauder, PhD, discovered that many women experience sharp, powerful orgasms as a result of the increased abdominal pressure of a full bladder.

★ Leave the other lubricants and gels in the bathroom cabinet. Most commercial jellies can be too lubricating and kill the friction needed for orgasm to happen. Use saliva or water instead.

★ You've already heard all the boring stuff about the virtues of a balanced diet – but if you eat right, your libido functions better. In particular, stock up on anything containing vitamin B (vegetables, eggs, nuts, brown rice and fruit) and zinc (fish, liver, mushrooms, red meat and grains), all of which will enhance the efficiency of the nervous system and hence lead to better orgasms.

★ For orgasmic pursuits, red-light booze. Alcohol dulls the nervous system, so while you might want him more after three Cosmopolitans, you'll get much less out of the proceedings.

★ A half-glass of red wine, on the other hand, will raise your testosterone levels and will make your reactions even more intense.

★ Speed things up with a double-sided approach. Sex researcher Shere Hite found that 70 per cent of women require clitoral stimulation in order to orgasm. So, combine a finger and a penis, a tongue and a finger, a vibrator and a tongue, then lay back and watch the explosions start!

★ Tobacco constricts the circulation of blood and may lower testosterone – the sex-drive hormone. Both of these are essential for an orgasm. A new study reveals that quitters had more orgasms afterwards than they did when they smoked.

★ Drink a coffee with two sugars. Since sugar and caffeine increase the heart rate and give a surge of energy, they can make your body more responsive to whatever nice things may be happening to it.

★ Ginseng has been shown to add spice to your orgasms, but make sure you choose your root carefully. Some of the cheaper brands have been shown to contain less than 10 per cent of the potent plant.

★ Orgasms aren't a basic instinct that we're born with – they're a learned talent that comes with practice.

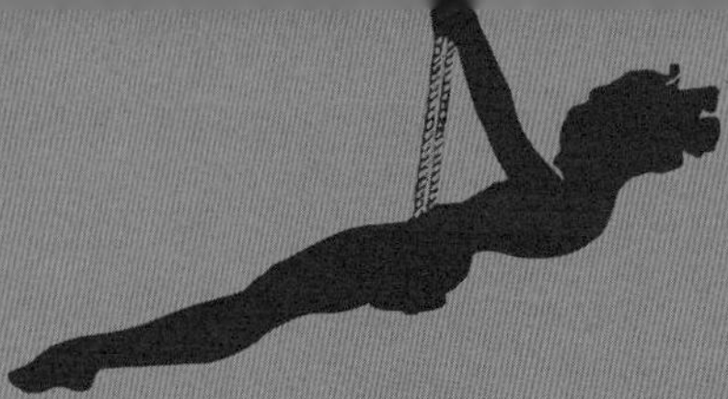

★ No two orgasms are alike for women. The climatic moment – supreme pleasure followed by a feeling of wellbeing and satisfaction – occurs in the brain's limbic system (or pleasure centre). Sensations can range from mild stimulation to an ecstasy so overwhelming that a woman momentarily loses consciousness. Recognize your range as opposed to going for an off-the-Richter Scale even, each and every time.

★ 53 per cent of men interviewed for *The Janus Report on Sexual Behaviour* replied that their partner's orgasmic pleasure was more important than their own, compared to only 34 per cent of women.

★ Between 10 per cent and 20 per cent of women have experienced a sleep orgasm. In that pleasurable experience, they are awakened by an erotic dream culminating in a climax. This is most likely to happen when you have been sexually deprived, but mentally stimulated. For example, he may be out of town, but not out of mind.

★ The average male orgasm lasts for10 to 30 seconds; the average female one is 13 to 51 seconds.

★ A rich meal eaten just before making love can inhibit orgasms.

★ Study or get promoted. One survey found that the two best predictors as to whether or not a woman would be able to reach orgasm during sex were education and social standing. Better-educated women with higher professional status were more likely to be orgasmic.

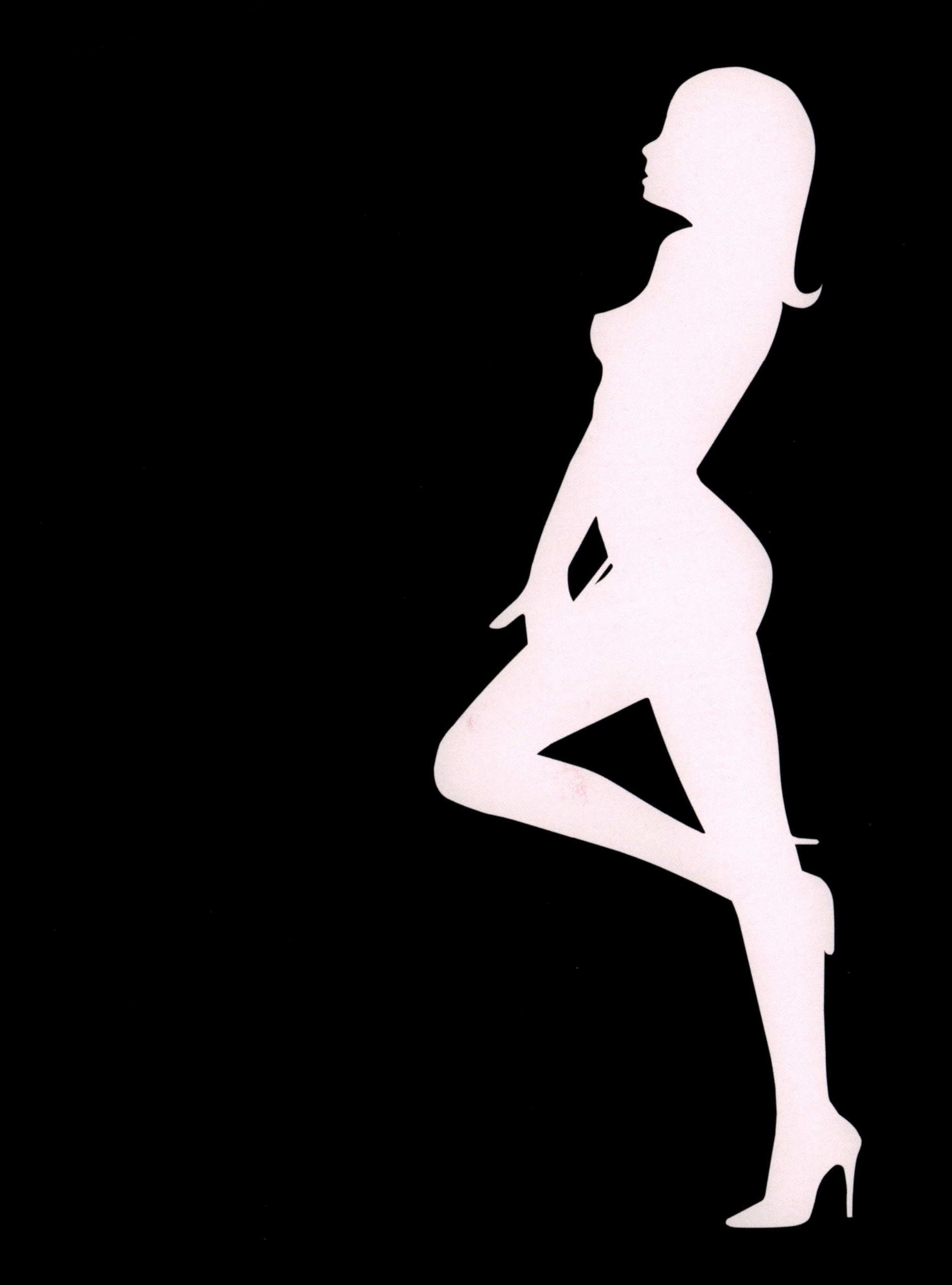

Orgasm Busts

Seven things can de-rail your pleasure. Here's how to get back on track...

PROBLEM: Breast-feeding – Prolactin, a hormone that produces breast milk, dampens your sex drive.
SOLUTION: Think about your baby. The hormone oxytocin, which releases milk into the breasts, also stimulates the contraction of the uterine muscles and may help a woman to climax.

PROBLEM: Stress – both cumulative and the daily 'stuck in traffic' kind – can lower testosterone and DHEA, a hormone that enhances sex drive and acts as a mood-booster.
SOLUTION: Before making love, take 20 minutes to re-group (take a walk, change into your playclothes or have a bath).

PROBLEM: Sleep deprivation. Women report that going to bed later than usual on one night can affect their libido the next evening. One possible reason why is that during slumber, levels of the stress hormone cortisol drop. Loss of sleep means that this hormone builds up and may erode a woman's wellbeing and possibly, her ability to experience sexual pleasure.
SOLUTION: Plan to get a full eight hours' sleep as soon as possible.

PROBLEM: The Pill – By suppressing ovulation, the Pill can lower levels of testosterone and inhibit desire.
SOLUTION: Work with your doctor to play with different levels of progesterone in your prescription.

PROBLEM: The room in which you're making love is illuminated with 175-watt light bulbs.
SOLUTION: Light some candles (but don't leave them unattended!)

PROBLEM: You feel self-conscious about your vaginal odour.
SOLUTION: Don't douche. Arousal gives your vagina its own natural muskiness. Look on it as your own custom-made sex perfume. (If it's really unpleasant, though, you may have picked up an infection and will need to get it checked out by a doctor.)

PROBLEM: You're scared you'll get pregnant or catch an STD (sexually-transmitted disease).
SOLUTION: Always use a condom. (You should do, anyway!)

PROBLEM: You've never had an orgasm.
SOLUTION: Get a blood test. Your anorgasmia (lack of orgasm) may be caused by an injury or abnormal growth on the anterior pituitary gland. Once the lesions are surgically removed, you'll soon become orgasmic.

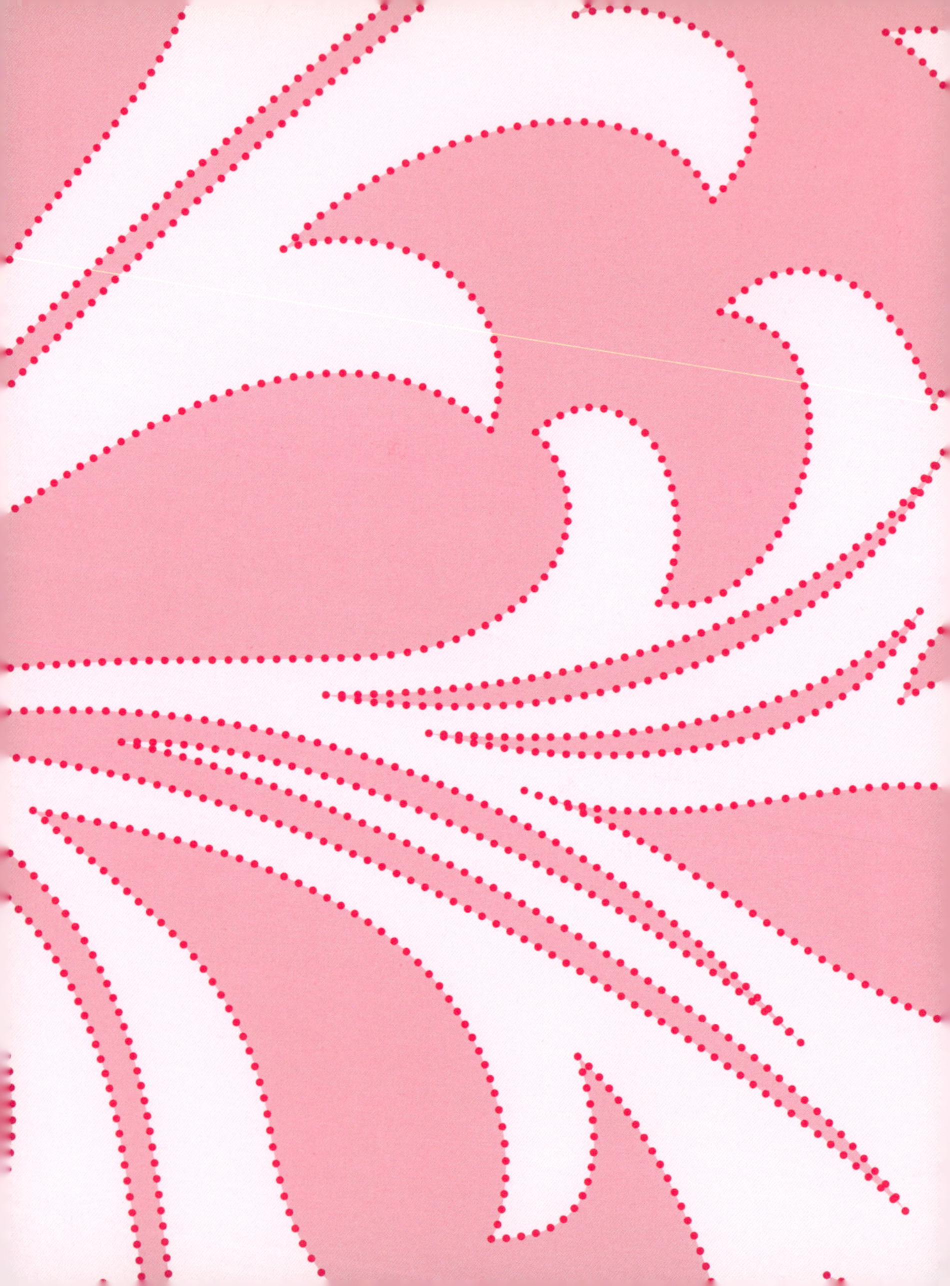

Chapter 5

Quickie Sex

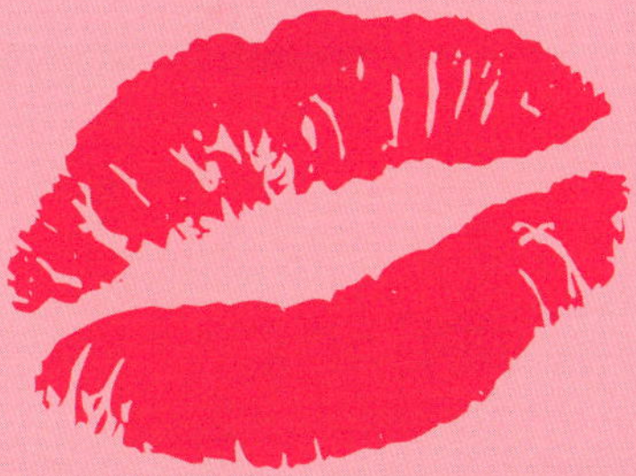

Minute One: On Your Mark

Let's face it, you're not always in the mood for some dreamy endless lovin'. Sometimes you're so damned hot you just want to fast forward past the Enya CD and the Tantric sex guidebooks and get on with the explosion.

The good news is that all it takes are five mad minutes to fire up your sex life big-time. That's right – 300 seconds. The fact is, there is nothing so exhilarating as fast, frenzied sex. Sex when you both have places to go, people to see, appointments to keep. Sex that is unplanned, impetuous and impulsive. Sex that borders on the forbidden or the foolhardy. Sex because you just have to have each other right here, right now.

Horny yet? Then leave the dishes. Be late for work. And hold on to your hats – your sex drive is about to zoom from zero to 60 in less time than it takes to read this page.

Seven Reasons to Do It Right Now

Having a quickie is essential for your mental health.

1 Stripped of all the trimmings, an orgasm is really just the physical release of built-up tension in the body. So quickies are a great way to de-stress (and much easier to get him to do than a massage).

2 Snagging a quickie is an instant mood lifter. Going fast and furious gets your blood flowing and boosts your endorphins for an oh-yeah booty bonus.

3 You jump-start your inner sex goddess by keeping your body pumped for action. According to research by Eileen Palace, PhD, the more stimulation your body receives, the more it is primed for being stimulated. So the more quickies you have, the more quickly you will get turned on.

4 A new way to spell relief: Q-U-I-C-K-I-E. According to research by Lawrence Robbins, MD, a dose of instant sex can help relieve women of pain from migraines (and it's a lot more energizing than a tranquillizer).

5 You're acting according to your biological nature. Humans were designed for fast sex, say evolutionary psychologists. The animal kingdom wasn't used to wasting time. The more time you spent copulating, the more vulnerable you were to being consumed by some woolly thing (and we don't mean your lover).

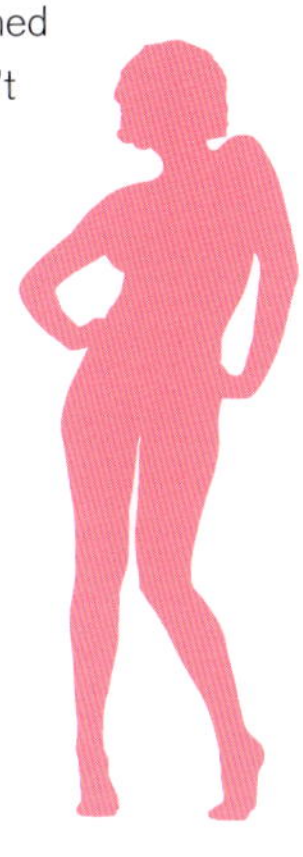

6 Quickies are efficient. They get the job done. So you get to have sex and still get a decent night's sleep at the end of it.

7 They're empowering. Yes, that's right. What could be more of a power trip than inciting your lover into a sexual frenzy?

Four Reasons He Wants You to Do It NOW

All it takes to plaster a goofy smile on his face is five minutes.

1 Men are suckers for a little mystery – studies show that the possibility of conquering the unknown is a top reason for why guys stray. Surprising him with some sex-on-the-run will stop him from thinking he knows all your secrets – keeping him as faithful as a St Bernard dog.

2 Research has found that an occasional quickie can be the answer to a lot of his sexual anxieties. There's no losing sleep over how long he has to last or whether he is giving you enough foreplay. All he has to do is get an erection and use it.

3 Some men – most men … OK … ALL men, at a certain level – have a weakness for rapid sex. It's fast, dirty and has a tinge of anonymity about it (according to a University of Vermont study, having sex with a stranger is his number one fantasy).

4 Two words: Minimal foreplay.

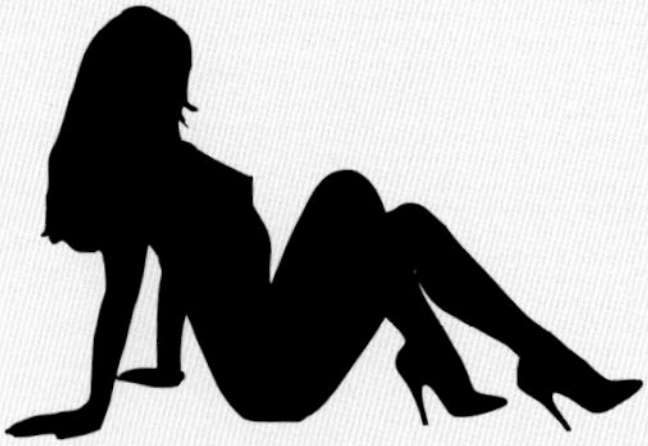

If You're Still Not Convinced

Seven MORE reasons why you really should do it right now – if only to have a more bonded union.

1 Who has the time or energy for all the prep work that goes into prolonged sex? Dimming the lights to a flattering glow, burning candles, bracing yourself for the never-ending G-spot expedition … yawn. Sex is like dining. Sure, the five-course gourmet deal is delicious. But sometimes, nothing but a hamburger will do.

2 Even a tired quickie can convey more tenderness than long hours of lovemaking. Bet this sounds familiar: You're exhausted. He wants sex. You love him so you don't want to reject him and you know you can do just about anything for five minutes.

3 While quickies may not be able to save a relationship in nosedive, they're certainly the easiest – and fastest – way to revive a boring sex life. If you're used to a certain method of making love, a fast body bash can break a ho-hum routine.

4 You'll keep the flames burning. Passion doesn't automatically keep going – you've got to work at it. The role of a quickie is to turn up the heat once in a while.

5 Quite simply, your relationship depends on it. According to a study by Ellen Bersheid, PhD, a psychologist who researches close relationships, in order for love to thrive, it's essential that lovers experience minor interruptions so that they can recapture an awareness of their emotional involvement. Because you've behaved unexpectedly and interrupted a pattern (that is, your usual Saturday night making-love-in-bed), he'll be reminded of how much he loves you.

6 Nano-second sex reminds both of you that there's always a little window of time to connect. (Three quickies a week is only 15 minutes. Anyone has time for that.)

7 The after-effects last a long, long time. One poll found that couples who regularly speed up sex, kiss, cuddle and hold hands more. How's that for afterplay?

So Not True

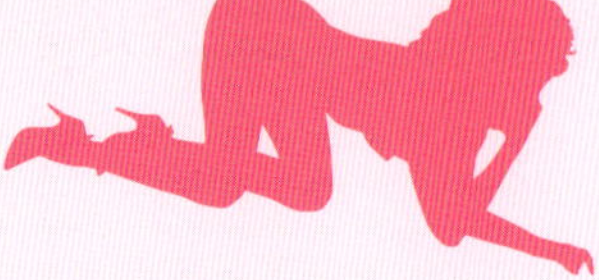

Take your time and read these quickie myths.

MYTH: Quickie sex bites.
TRUTH: Arousal is a mysterious and powerful thing, so the frantic abandon of a quick fix can ignite a climax that's every bit as explosive as a marathon session in the sack.

MYTH: Women need at least 72 hours of foreplay to have an orgasm.
TRUTH: Actually, cutting to the chase sexually can pay off passionately for both of you. The evidence shows that we don't exactly need a lot of time to experience sexual nirvana – according to studies by sex researchers Carol Darling, PhD, and Kenneth Davidson, women can, on average, reach orgasm in eight minutes with a partner. In other words, full-blown, drawn-out foreplay, while tasty, is really just additional sauce.

MYTH: Women hate quickies.
TRUTH: *Au contraire.* In one survey conducted by Bowling Green State University, a group of men and women, aged between 25 and 43, were asked, 'If you had to make one choice – and you could have only one – which would you choose: hard, driving fast sex or slow, gentle sex?' The majority of the women wanted to get hammered.

MYTH: Languorous lovemaking, hours in bed, kisses and caresses that go on forever and back rubs are necessary for good sex.
TRUTH: You can be TOO relaxed. According to a Tulane University study, since orgasm is a tension release, the more stirred you are mentally during sex, the higher your bliss potential.

MYTH: If he wants a quickie, it means he doesn't love you.
TRUTH: Every act of sex doesn't have to be a relationship seminar. Studies show that couples who don't mind doing it quickly every once in a while have MORE sex because they don't place so much emphasis behind the meaning of each carnal moment together.

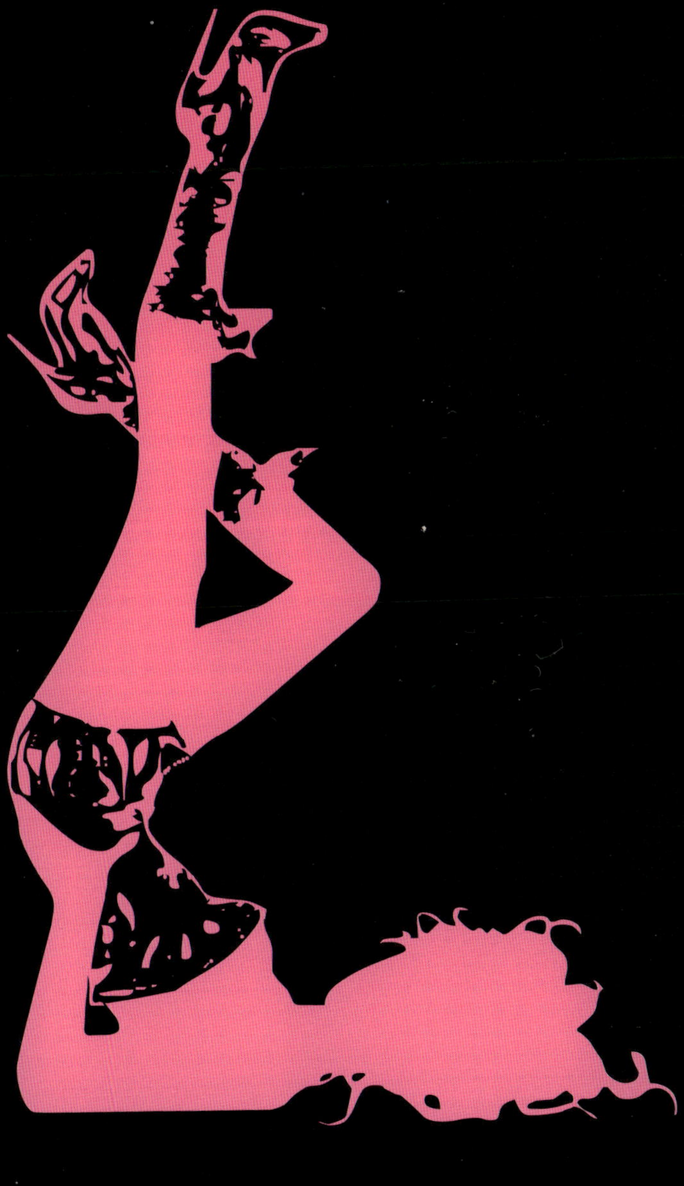

Minute Two: Get Ready

True, the great thing about a quickie is that it's pretty much a no-frills, anything goes proposition. There's no obsessing about setting the perfect mood, wearing the right lingerie or putting on clean sheets. For that matter, who needs sheets at all?

But the reality is that sex never happens spontaneously. If you expect it to, you're setting yourself up for disappointment. Generally, there's always a prelude that leads us to be sexual, say sex experts. A certain loving touch, a special outfit that gets us in the mood. Bottom line: whatever our preliminaries, we never come cold to sex, we always prepare. So here are a few fast-and-loose guiding principles to prep you for chasing the World's Fastest Orgasm title. What are you waiting for?

One Minute to Better Whoa!

Learn to exercise control.

Limber your love muscles. According to the American Association of Sex Educators, Counsellors and Therapists, toning your pubococcygeus (PC) muscles helps lubricate and stimulate you, making your orgasms come on more quickly and more intensely (this goes for men, too). No one will know what you're doing, so go ahead and squeeze when you're stuck in a traffic jam, you're bored at work or getting your hair done.

1 Find the right muscles – the ones you use to stop your urine flow.
2 Exercise them – squeeze and hold tight for three seconds. Relax for three seconds, then repeat, building up until you can maintain a squeeze for ten seconds. The more you do, the stronger the results.

BONUS: Squeezing those PC muscles makes you aware of your vagina and clitoris, sending little turn-on messages to your body. To use during sex, squeeze as he slides out and release as he plunges in. It'll feel like a suction cup around his penis and create tantalizing friction for both of you.

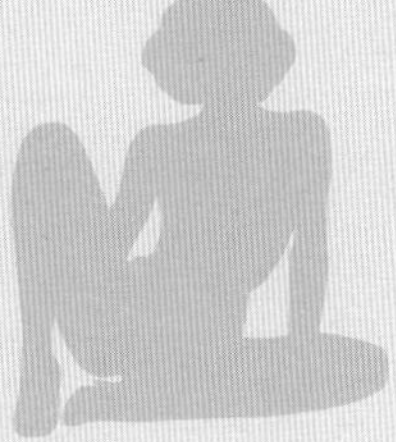

A-Sex-Orize

How to dress for the occasion.

★ Plan on staying semi-clothed. If you're prepared to get naked, you're not impatient enough to get into the swing of the quickie. Of course, ripping your clothes off is a different story.

★ Wear a suspender (garter) belt to work, you naughty thing. It'll give him easy access later.

★ Slip into something new. According to one survey, husbands who fail to notice that their wives changed their hair colour from black to blonde literally leapt to attention at the sight of a fresh-off-the-rack pair of lace underpants or an unfamiliar push-up bra.

★ You don't have time to worry about your body during a quickie. So disguise your jelly belly with big panties that cut just above the belly button and make your stomach look flatter, a more practical solution than sucking in your breath.

★ Forget fashion and slip into a longish, loose skirt – it's ideal for hiking up and making a quick discreet connection in public places.

★ If you can't skip underwear altogether, make them edible.

★ A sexy teddy or leotard that opens at the crotch will have you ready in a snap.

★ Y-fronts or boxer shorts for him were designed with a quickie in mind.

Introduce a Third Party

There's nothing like your own personal joystick to get a buzz in a flash.

★ A Magic Wand vibrator, with a ball-shaped vibrating head, flexible neck and long cylindrical body is best for both of you (available online from www.annsummers.com).

★ Using a battery-operated vibrator will ensure that you don't run out of steam mid-play. According to the sex toy store Good Vibrations (www.goodvibes.com), the best are Japanese-made.

★ Best high-speed move: Press your new love toy against (not on) your clitoris or insert it into your vagina. Run it along the bottom side of the penis. Indirect vibes create a deeper, more satisfying orgasm than ones that hit your bulls-eye.

★ Woman-on-top and rear-entry positions allow plenty of room to get a good buzz going.

★ Pressing the head of the vibrator against your tummy will make you arch with ecstasy.

Hurry-Up Helps

Tricks to heat the action up in a flash.

★ Eat right. Chocolate contains phenylethylamine, a mood-boosting chemical that can incite lust. Oysters are a good source of zinc, which studies show help his standing-to-attention powers. Other research suggests that seafood in general, which is high in protein, is also high in tyrosine, an amino acid that can act as a libido pick-you-up. And chilli peppers trigger the release of endorphins, feel-good brain chemicals that make you ready for action.

★ Get wet. Studies by sex researchers John Wincze, PhD, and Patricia Schriener-Engel, PhD, have shown our body's responses sometimes take time to catch up with our mental urges. Adding a drop of water-based lubricant to the head of the penis (or condom) before sex will keep your body and mind on the same sexy wavelength.

★ Forget crooners like Luther Vandross and Natalie Cole. A study from Loyola University discovered that heavy metal and other hard-rock variations get his pulses (and other bits) racing. So make sure you have a Limp Bizkit or Linkin Park CD in your collection.

★ Stick your schnoz in his underarm. A recent Bern University study found that this is where a whiff of someone's scent can send you into a sexual frenzy. A sniff of lavender and pumpkin pie will have the same stiffening effect on him – the Scent Smell and Taste Treatment and Research Foundation in Chicago discovered that these combined odours increase penile blood flow by 40 per cent.

★ Come – er – prepared. Studies on easily orgasmic women (those who climax more than 90 per cent of the time) have found that they often anticipate steamy encounters hours – even days – before (see page 137 for suggestions).

★ You knew there had to be a good reason you were logging all those hours in tush-tightening class. A University of Washington study found a quick 20-minute workout primes our bodies for sex (and not just because we're at the gym ogling sweaty, buff men doing bench presses). It seems a hard-pumping heart sends blood to all extremities – including sex organs. So pump your own iron before you pump his.

★ Bump up your secret hot spot. Build sexual tension with this indirect pleasure prep: massage the area about one middle finger length below your belly button. Pressing it gently for about three minutes helps promote blood flow, firing up the whole pelvic area.

★ Keep a naked snap of your man (or anything you think looks really sexy) in your wallet. You'll feel flirty all day.

★ Carry a quickie kit: Keep condoms, any props like scarves or handcuffs (for a little light bondage), lubrication and a compact mirror and hairbrush (for post-sex sprucing) to hand, so that in the midst of passion, you don't get stalled on technicalities.

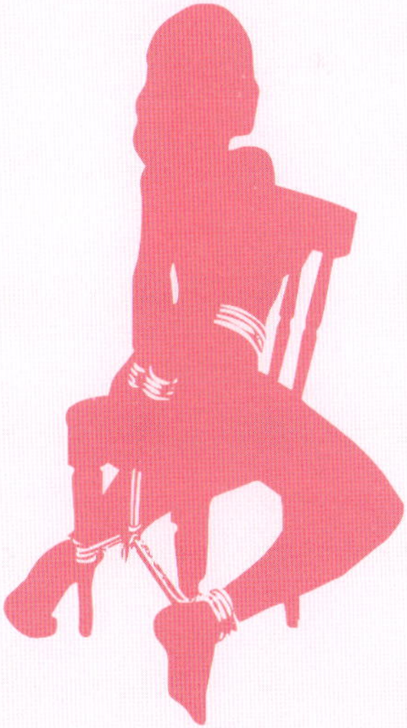

Pick-You-Uppers

Fuel up with the following to turn your libido into Speedy Gonzales.

★ According to studies, fish and beans can turn his wood from willow to mahogany.

★ Take a daily dose of libido-boosting homeopathic remedies like graphite, lycopodium or pulsatilla and say, 'Hubba-hubba'.

★ Red wine boosts testosterone levels to make your reactions raunchier – especially if you're on the Pill.

★ Give yourself an energy boost. Vitamin C energy powders will give you the orgasmic stamina you need for a quickie.

★ Get a buzz on with bee pollen. Research shows that it lifts energy levels, libido, sexual potency and fertility. How sweet it is!

★ Spicy foods such as chillies, garlic and onions ignite sexual passion. Just make sure you carry breath mints with you!

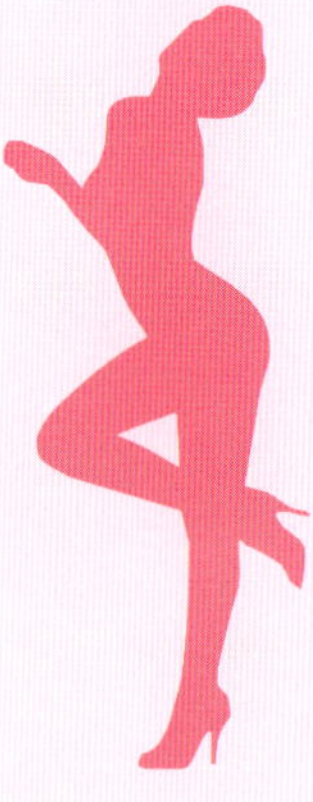

Hot and Bothered

Give him THAT sign.

★ Simply take his fingers and put them in your mouth. It will send an instant message to his groin.

★ Get right to the point – lift up your top and press your cleavage against his back.

★ Try blinking in time to his breathing – it's like flashing the word SEX in front of his eyes.

★ Place his hands where you want them – on you.

★ Create a quickie code, perhaps a wink or a secret handshake that says in no uncertain terms 'You, me, here, now', to preclude any awkward misunderstandings or long, boring waits in the bathroom for an unwitting partner.

★ Stare directly at his crotch.

★ When you're out in a public place, disappear for a few minutes then, when you return, hand him your panties. Or whisper that you are wearing edible panties in his ear.

★ Greet him naked.

Minute Three: Get Set

Here's a newsflash: he doesn't hold a patent on horniness. It seems that both men and women have a supply of the hormones that propel the sex drive into amorous action: oestrogen, progesterone and testosterone.

But there's more to keeping your sex drive in gear than pushing the right buttons or putting a tiger in your tank. To have all the heady force of a turbocharged engine in peak performance, your sex drive has to be revved emotionally as well as physically. That goes for men as well as women.

Here, then, is the owner's manual for getting your mind and body focused back to where it damn well should be – sex! Your car mechanic may not know about them, but these aids are a sure-fire guarantee for ignition.

Mental Hurdles

Having an orgasm is often 80 per cent mental and 20 per cent physical. Here's how to get in the right state of mind to enter the Oh! zone.

★ Sex up your brain. Fantasize or watch something sexy to get you in the mood (log on to www.nerve.com if you don't have any steamy video tapes to hand).

★ Have a few drinks. While studies show that booze inhibits men, it actually has the opposite effect on women (as long as you keep it to two).

★ Think you are enjoying yourself and you will. Even if it feels as if you're just going through the motions at first, it will feel great in just a minute. According to studies by sex researcher Eileen Palace, PhD, when women raise their expectations about sex (and think, 'of course my toes will curl'), their bodies become more responsive within 30 seconds.

★ Get over it. Sex doesn't cure cancer. It also doesn't ensure world peace or bring down Superpowers. The point is, getting it right every time isn't that important. If you start fretting about whether you'll break sexual records, just start repeating to yourself: 'This feels good, this feels good' – in other words, forcing your mind to go with the flow.

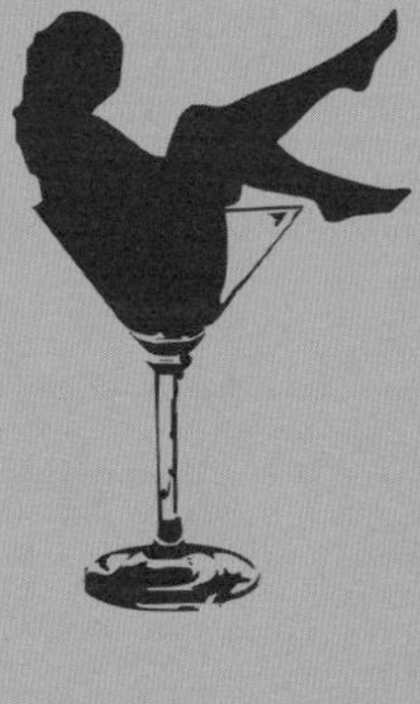

Master Your Own Domain

Give yourself a helping hand to remain in a sex-ready state.

★ When masturbating, women do not linger any longer than men: Kinsey reported that it takes an average of about three minutes for both to come to orgasm.

★ Studies have found that the erotic highs from masturbation can last a few hours. So you can speed things up by letting your fingers do the walking long before your lover arrives on the scene.

★ In one poll, 95 per cent of men said they like it when their lover creates her own pleasure. On one hand, it takes the pressure off them. On the other, it's just plain hot.

★ Wet your fingers first.

★ Locate the target: Touching the clitoris directly may be too intense, which means that instead of building up to an orgasm you may feel numbness or even pain. To avoid this, press your index and middle fingers on either side of outer lips, gently squeezing the fingers together in a circular motion to stimulate the clitoral ridge underneath.

★ Squeezing and contracting your thigh muscles while thrusting helps massage your clitoris against his hard body.

A Quickie Fix

Bed-tested techniques guaranteed to make the earth move in sync.

YOU'RE HOT, HE'S NOT: The quickest way to get a man hard is to go straight to the heart of the matter: his penis (a Pirelli calendar nearby doesn't hurt either). Three tips: use a firm grip, a wet hand and flick your tongue.

HE'S HOT, YOU'RE NOT: You can waste time with him poking here and prodding there. But no one knows how to warm you up better than little ol' you. A little spit or lubrication on the finger will speed things along. Put your hand over his to make him putty in your hands.

HE NEEDS TO SLOW DOWN: According to the Kinsey Institute clock, a man can go from start to finish in one minute. To pace himself to last another 120 seconds, he can:

♥ Flex his muscles (when a man contracts his PCs – direct his attention to page 129 – he can lower arousal a few notches).
♥ Breathe deeply (it directs blood away from his penis).
♥ Open his legs (when he is lying on top, he can spread his legs to take the pressure off his testicles – when they are too compressed, they become overstimulated.
♥ Change gears (simply changing positions can halt his momentum).
♥ Take it out (it removes him from the seat of action – blowing warm air onto it will keep him hot without exciting him to the point of no return).

YOU NEED TO SPEED UP: Once a woman is hot, she can keep pace with any man. The trick is getting to the race on time:

♥ Let him help you get a head start with a one-minute visit south of the border (studies show oral sex has the double bonus of quickly lubricating and stimulating you in all the right places).
♥ Give yourself a helping hand (see Master Your Own Domain, opposite).
♥ Position yourself correctly (getting on top will help his penis connect with your clitoris while rear entry is best suited for hands-on sex).

Minute Four: Go!

With time at a premium, we're going to cut to the chase. Here, handy tips for doing the horizontal indoors, outdoors and everywhere in between.

Yes, it's risky. That's precisely the point. Moderate fear – not staring-down-an-agitated-lion fear but the kind you feel when you could potentially be caught doing something naughty – causes the production of adrenaline, the sexy pick-me-up you manufacture when you're aroused. But exercise discretion. While the other half of the thrill of a quickie is that the world, so to speak, is your mattress, you can be fined or arrested if caught.

Get Your Timing Right

When it comes to catching the orgasm express, timing is everything.

Skip lunch and have a nooner instead. Testosterone levels in adult males are subject to circadian rhythms, researchers have found, meaning that they rise and fall in 24-hour cycles – and they tend to peak shortly before 12 pm.

Your body starts screaming yes, yes, yes around mid-cycle (14 days after your last period) when oestrogen levels are at their highest.

Don't do it: hold off having sex for two weeks and it'll add instant heat to your flash-in-the-pan coupling.

Make a quickie your wake-up call. It's better than an alarm and the chances are, he'll already be hard.

Location, Location, Location

Any where, any time, any place.

CONCRETE JUNGLE

Unless you're a masochist, if you're romping in an alley or on a road, you'll want minimal ground contact.

- ♥ For a raunchy position that stops your clothes from getting dirty and your bottom getting cold, he should squat on his heels while you sit on his upper thighs facing him with your weight on your feet. Wrap your arms around him for balance.
- ♥ Another hot move: Stand facing the wall with your feet about 45 cm (18 in) apart. Standing facing your back with his feet between yours, he bends his knees and enters you from below. Holding your hips to steady himself, he leans back while you lean forwards against wall, his hips pressed against your hips.

ON THE MOVE

Live life in the fast lane.

- ♥ Do it on a roller coaster. Studies show that screaming your head off on a ride causes a surge in adrenaline and endorphins, both of which give you a sexy thrill.
- ♥ The seat belts in your car can be used for light bondage at a pinch.
- ♥ Inside the car, avoid unintentional pressing of the horn during the throes of abandonment (drawing embarrassing attention to the vehicle) by jumping into the back seat. Another good car position is him sitting in the passenger seat with you on his lap facing him (if your legs are very long, you can rest them on his shoulders).
- ♥ It's easy to hide a hand job under one of those little airplane blankets. And if you're really sneaky, you can rest your head on your partner's lap and just happen to have oral sex. But try not to let your head bob up and down (unless there's turbulence).
- ♥ Join the Mile High Club (then you can register at www.milehighclub.com) by having sex on a plane once you reach cruising altitude. You can make a quick getaway to the toilet during the movie when there's usually no meal or beverage services. Face-to-face standing sex is best or he can enter you from behind (BONUS: you can both watch in the mirror).

H2-OHHH!

Make your own waves.

- ♥ Hold on to your bikini bottoms. You don't want to do the 'walk of shame' back to your towel.
- ♥ The perfect pool or ocean water level is waist high (any lower and it's embarrassing, any higher and your passion may be swept away). If you're surrounded by sunbathers, hold your breath and sink to the bottom, pull your bikini bottoms to one side and let him perform oral thrill.
- ♥ Have him stand up and enter you while you float on your back – now try that when you're landlocked!
- ♥ In general, the water needs to be quite warm so his erection won't sink. However, the heat in a hot tub can cause blood vessels to dilate so his erection may not be as firm.
- ♥ While the beach seems movie-made for getting swept away, when sand gets in the creases and holds of the vagina, it can cause abrasions (think sandpaper), which makes it easier to catch STDs, including HIV.
- ♥ If possible, have him enter you before you get wet and wild so your natural wetness doesn't wash away first.

GOING GREEN

Become a nature lover.

- ♥ Make use of the great outdoors. Sunlight is additive-free Viagra. One theory is that it makes people hornier because it suppresses their melatonin, a hormone believed to be the biological version of a five-course meal (in other words, it diminishes sexual desire). At the same time, it's speculated that sunshine increases serotonin and other hormones that make us more open to back-to-nature nookie.
- ♥ Do it in a cucumber patch – according to a study conducted by the Smell and Taste Treatment and Research Foundation, the most arousing smell for women is cucumber (lavender comes in second, great if you're in Provence).
- ♥ If passion overtakes you while you're walking in the woods, remember that mozzies love moist dark places – you get the picture (ouch!). Spray yourselves with repellent before heading out. A blanket or sleeping bag will also serve as barrier between you and any creepy crawlies.

- ♥ Make sure you know what stinging nettles and poison ivy look like (check out a website like www.vth.colostate.edu/poisonous_plants).
- ♥ If you want extra wood, choose a tree wider than your hips so it'll hold you up as you lean back against it. If the bark is smooth, you can prop your bottom against it and wrap your legs around his waist so that it supports your weight.

ON THE TOWN

Make a break for it.

- ♥ Hit the bathroom when you're at a restaurant. The locked door won't arouse suspicion for at least five minutes (which is all you need). Also watching yourselves in the mirror as you go at it is pretty damned hot.
- ♥ Go for the ladies' toilet, as there is more privacy there than in the gents'.
- ♥ If you do it in a dressing room, be careful about doing it against shoddy walls (they may collapse). A changing bench or chair is much easier and won't arouse the suspicion of any curious salespeople.
- ♥ You can have a quickie without leaving your table at a restaurant if the tablecloth is long. Just use your big toe to masturbate each other.
- ♥ At the office, use a chair without wheels and flick on the computer monitor for sexy mood lighting (he sits and you perch on his lap).
- ♥ If you're at a boring party, head for a tight closet. He can squat on his knees while you lay on your back resting your knees on your chest and placing your feet on his torso. Start your motors. It's easy to get into and you get lots of deep thrusting.

Get in Position

The top moves to master for playing beat-the-clock sex.

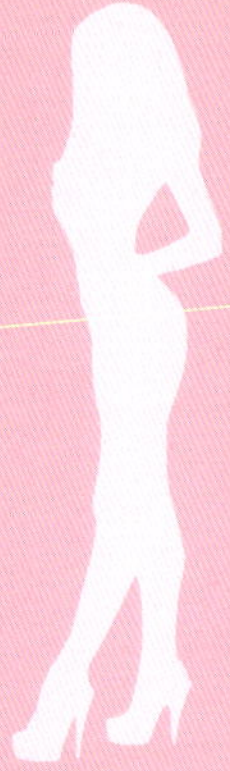

STANDING UP

- It can be tricky to match up your love organs if you're different heights, so face away from him and bend over so that your hands are flat on the floor and your weight is forwards (or lean against a wall). He simply enters you from behind. Because all you have to do is slip down your knickers (or just wear crotchless), you can take this show on the road – your office desk, the restaurant toilet, wherever the urge strikes.
- Doing it on the stairs will also even things out.
- If he's strong and you're light, try what the Kama Sutra calls 'suspended congress': while he leans back against a wall, you face him, sitting on his joined-together hands (he should lace his fingers), with your arms around his neck. You can move yourself by extending your legs and putting your feet against the wall.

SOME MOVES ARE TWO-IN-ONE

- Anything rear entry gives the deep penetration often needed with quick sex and lets his penis hit the ultrasensitive front of your vaginal wall.
- If you're sitting in a chair, face away from him, as he can then also massage your clitoris. Hooking your leg over the chair leg will create extra friction between your clitoris and his penis.
- Keep your legs together: This straight-laced position can trigger an instant orgasm by making it easier to clench your thigh muscles, which continue far up enough to stimulate your inner clitoris (the tissue actually extends 9 cm (3.5 in) – about the length of your middle finger – up into the pelvic area).
- Wear a girdle – sexy – yes! It puts pressure on the lower abs, which stimulates your inner clitoris (see above). Or get him to use his hand – anything that presses down on the part of your abs just above your pubic mound (his hand, your hand, a stack of bricks) during intercourse should do the trick because it sandwiches your inner clitoris between the proverbial rock and a hard place – in this case, your tensed muscles and his penis. Extra tip – make sure he's inside you first as it will be difficult for him to hit the mark otherwise.

THE DOOR JAMB

Make use of the entryways to both your body and home with this position (part of the appeal is you may get busted by neighbours or flat-mates). Caution: don't wear socks, it can make things uncomfortably slippery. Find a narrow doorway. He leans backwards against the door jamb while you do the same with the other, straddling him. You can figure out the rest.

THE ONE-MINUTE

So-called because that's all he'll be able to hold it for unless he's Arnie Schwarzenegger. He sits down with his legs bent and his feet flat on the floor and his hands on the ground behind him. He pushes his bottom up off the floor, supporting his weight with his arms and legs. You mount, crouching over him, and ride off into the sunset.

Home Sweet Home

Listen to your mother's advice: Get out of bed!

- Have sex sitting on or leaning against a washing machine during the spin cycle for an extra orgasmic spin.
- The nozzle at your kitchen sink will add new meaning to the phrase, 'getting hosed' when used during a quickie.
- Handy for sex in the kitchen or any other confined space is sitting face-to-face and wrapping your legs around his waist and your arms around his neck.
- If you stop on the stairs, stand one step higher to make penetration a snap.
- Straight-back chairs give more room for manoeuvring. You can sit on his lap facing away from him or wrap your legs around him facing him. Or kneel on the chair holding onto the back (though you may topple over if things get vigorous – which we hope they will).

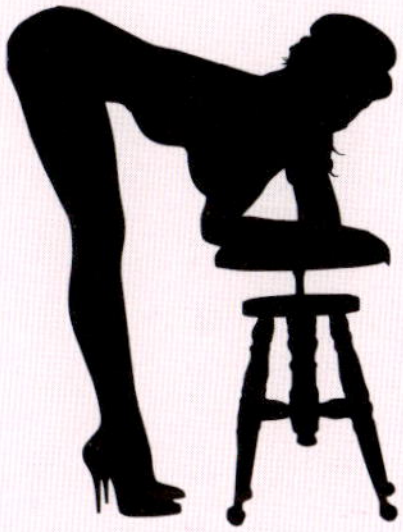

Minute Five: Oh!

You might think that all it takes to have a quickie is a penis, a vagina and a few minutes. Not so fast.

Here is something you don't know: Erogenous zones – dense nerve endings – crackle all over the body, particularly in the earlobes, neck, palms, inner thighs and the backs of the knees. In one study, women were able to orgasm simply from having their arms stroked.

Men's and women's bodies have roughly the same landscape of nerve endings, meaning there's a whole continent of hot spots out there for the taking. The quickie is ideally suited for starting your pleasure expedition. Since you need to move quickly, here's your love map for increasing your thrill power in a hurry. Get ready to spin your orgasms into roargasms.

Just Do It

New five-second tricks for packing 30 minutes of lovemaking into five.

TALK DIRTY: Tell your lover what you want. Explicitly. Some suggestions: 'Mmm, squeeze my nipple. Harder. Yes, that feels so good' – and so on. You get the idea. This isn't just to turn him on (though that's definitely a blissful side effect). But according to a Journal of Sex and Marital Therapy study, women who can talk freely about sex have a higher degree of sexual satisfaction than those who can't. Now that should get you saying 'Yes, yes, yes!'

GO FOR HIS JUGULAR: There is evidence that the physiological state of sexual arousal is similar to the physiological stress state of fear, anxiety or threat. In each of these states, blood pressure rises, the pulse quickens, adrenaline is released into the system and the body is energized and alert. Physically, the body is primed, and it may be possible to transform that primed state into a frenzy of sexual excitement.

BE SELFISH: Remember all that stuff your mother taught you about being polite? Forget it. This is no time to worry about the other guy. A quickie is every man and woman for himself and herself in a mad thrash for ecstasy. If you're thinking about pleasing him or he's thinking about satisfying you, then you're both missing the point. Don't think about anything except giving yourself pleasure.

ACCORDING TO ONE POLL, 40 per cent of men questioned are turned gooey by the natural scent of your nether regions. Not surprising since your vagina is a potent source of pheromones, chemicals that attract the opposite sex. Use it to your advantage – touch your vagina and bring the scent to your partner's nose for a guaranteed turn-on.

USE YOUR EYES AS WELL AS YOUR HANDS AND MOUTH. A 1986 Archives of Sexual Behavior study reveals that both men and women are stimulated by erotic images, so keep the lights on and your eyes wide open.

PUMP UP HIS PASSION by playing him a subliminally sensual tape of his favourite tunes. Music actually activates the pleasure circuits of the brain – the response can be so strong that it can even be orgasmic, according to a McGill University study on the subject.

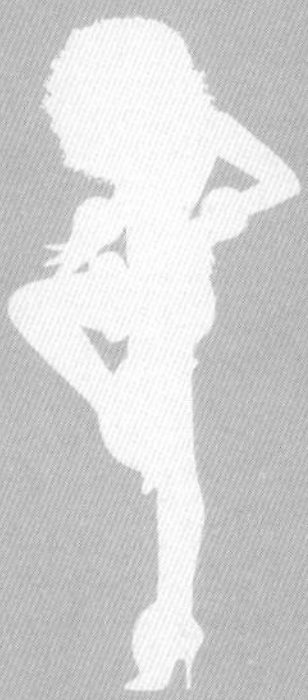

BECOME A LADY IN RED. The colour crimson is reputed to amp up passion and enthusiasm, so wear it when you want some feel-good fire.

Let Your Fingers Do the Walking

To make the most of your time, here are a few pointers to keep at your (and his) fingertips.

TEMPLES: Press your partner's temples and you'll feel veins throbbing. This pleasure point seems to have a direct link with the hypothalamus, your brain's bliss centre.

EARS: The cliché of blowing in your lover's ear is dead-on accurate. Stimulation from a darting tongue or a light, probing finger is such a powerful aphrodisiac that it can bring some men to orgasm. Researchers call the phenomenon the auriculogenital reflex and trace its origins to a nerve in the ear canal.

MOUTH: Trace the outline of your partner's lips. He'll feel a familiar zing when you reach the comer of his mouth. This area is packed with rarely reached nerves just longing for some good loving.

NECK AND SPINE: Try quick, playful love bites, especially on the ultra-sensitive collarbone. Move towards the centre of the back and trace the contours of the spine lightly with your tongue. Travel up and down your partner's back, blowing and tickling lightly as you go and watch him arch with pleasure.

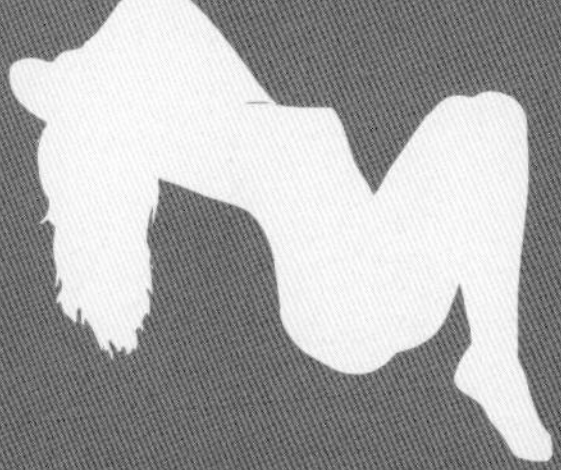

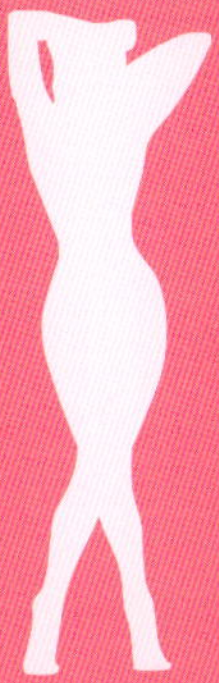

UNDERARMS: The tremendous accumulation of nerve endings here makes for great erotic potential. For a go-weak-at-the-knees move, use only your fingertips to stroke lightly and rhythmically from the rib cage towards the arms.

NIPPLES: You know that yours like attention, but so do his. Researchers have discovered that men's breasts have the same potential for erotic pleasure as women's breasts. In both sexes, the breasts are richly supplied with nerve endings, especially in the nipple area. Although only half as many men as women get hard nipples spontaneously when aroused, men's nipples are about as likely as women's to become erect when directly stimulated, and the sensation can sometimes make him explode.

BELLY BUTTON: Anthropologists call it a 'genital echo', meaning its shape reminds us of the vaginal opening, turning it into an instant visual turn-on. Heighten the pleasure by probing it with a darting tongue while tracing the outline with your index finger.

INNER THIGHS: This patch of land is ablaze with nerve endings because of the proximity to the genitals. Start with strokes so light that they barely register on your fingertips, and build to a crescendo of long, powerful strokes that work your fingers deep into the tender thigh muscles. Wowza.

FINGERS AND TOES: Yes, it's true. Suck away. And don't forget to use your tongue to probe the crevices between each and every digit (on second thought, this might be best when in water – see page 142 – to keep things spic 'n span).

Going Downtown

Measure for measure the muscle in your mouth holds more potential for pleasure than the one between your legs (and that goes for him, too).

★ Take a sip of water to keep your mouth – and things – wet and shiny.

★ Vary the temperature: Sip a hot drink or keep an ice cube in your mouth.

★ To speed things up, let your mouth and hands work together.

★ The flavour of your sexual marinade depends on your diet: Cow chompers have a pungent zest, vegetarians have a subtler flavour, spice lovers will pack a potent punch and the booze and ciggie brigade will have a slightly sour taste.

★ Hum.

★ Men tend to use their tongues like a mini penis. Instead, give him a new mental image with three words: 'ice scream' cone.

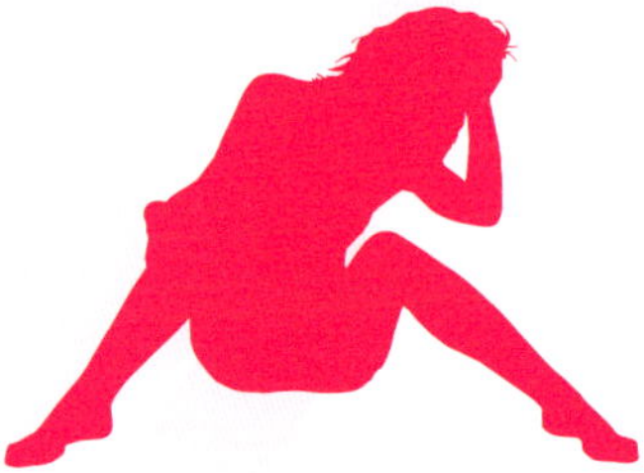

A Direct Hit

Ultimately, you will need to focus – these sex-marks-the-spots are guaranteed to get your erotic juices flowing.

WAYS TO WORK HIS PENIS:

- ♥ Don't rush when giving him a hand-job. Going at warp speed will sometimes kill the sensation for him, so take it down a notch (in the time it takes to say 'Mississippi', you should go up and down about two times).
- ♥ Most women use a simple up-and-down stroke with the thumb pointing up for a hand-job. Instead, start with the thumb pointing down and stroke up. When you get to the head, flip your hand over and go down. Then switch to the other hand.
- ♥ The V-Spot: There's a V-shaped break in the ridge that runs around the head of his penis – this is a small patch of skin can bring mind-blowing bliss (just think of him stroking your clitoris).
- ♥ The blood vessel-like seam on the underside of his penis that runs from just below the shaft to halfway down the scrotum is his scream seam. Massaging it will directly massage his urethra – a super-sensitive tube that is capable of registering intense pleasure.

HERE'S HOW TO MAKE IT HAPPEN EVERY TIME

- ♥ ON HIM: Poke his perineum (the thumbnail-sized dimple just behind his scrotum).
- ♥ ON YOU: Clitoris, clitoris, clitoris – like the estate agents say, it's all about location. But there are also points inside the vagina that get hot when pressed – the G-spot (one-third of the way up the canal on the front wall), the AFE zone (another third up – stimulation of this spot also helps lubrication and sometimes leads to multiple orgasms) and the cervix (the lump-like opening to the uterus at the end of the canal).

Speed Busters

You can go from 1,000 to less than zero on the thrillometre in less time than it takes to say, 'Ouch'. Since you may not have time to restart your play, here's what to avoid in the first place.

★ Not kissing first. Avoiding the lips and diving straight for the erogenous zones gives the experience a pay-by-the-hour feeling where you're trying to get your money's worth by cutting out nonessentials. Of course, this may be the effect you're going for.

★ Breaking contact. The biggest downer to having a quickie is the lack of intimacy. Always keeping in touch with your partner's body makes a big difference. Move your hands together, or stroke them one at a time, in a continual flow. If you have to stop, keep one hand gently resting against your partner's body.

★ Not taking the extra minute to get hot and sweaty.

★ Yes, there's hammering. But you can still go too hard. If he bashes his hip bones into your thigh or stomach, the pain is equal to two weeks of strenuous exercise concentrated into a few seconds.

★ Positioning yourselves incorrectly. The missionary position limits your clitoral stimulation, as well as your ability to move around beneath his body.

★ Giving a wedgie during foreplay. Stroking gently through panties can be very sexy. Pulling the material up between the thighs and yanking it back and forth in your rush to get on with the action is not.

★ Getting a non-battery powered vibrator (you don't want to waste precious minutes looking for a convenient outlet).

★ Forgetting, in your haste, to use any birth control.

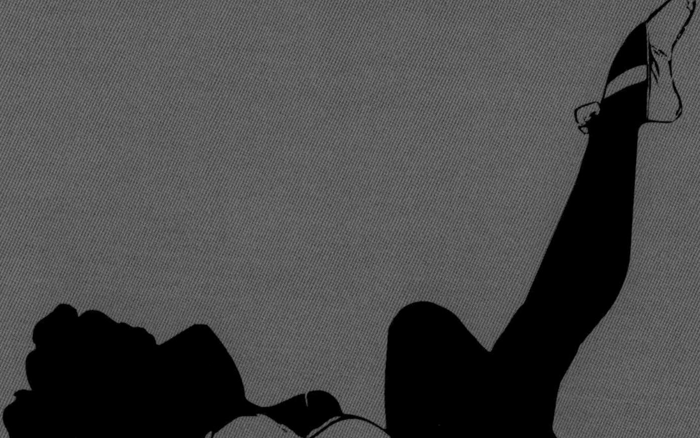

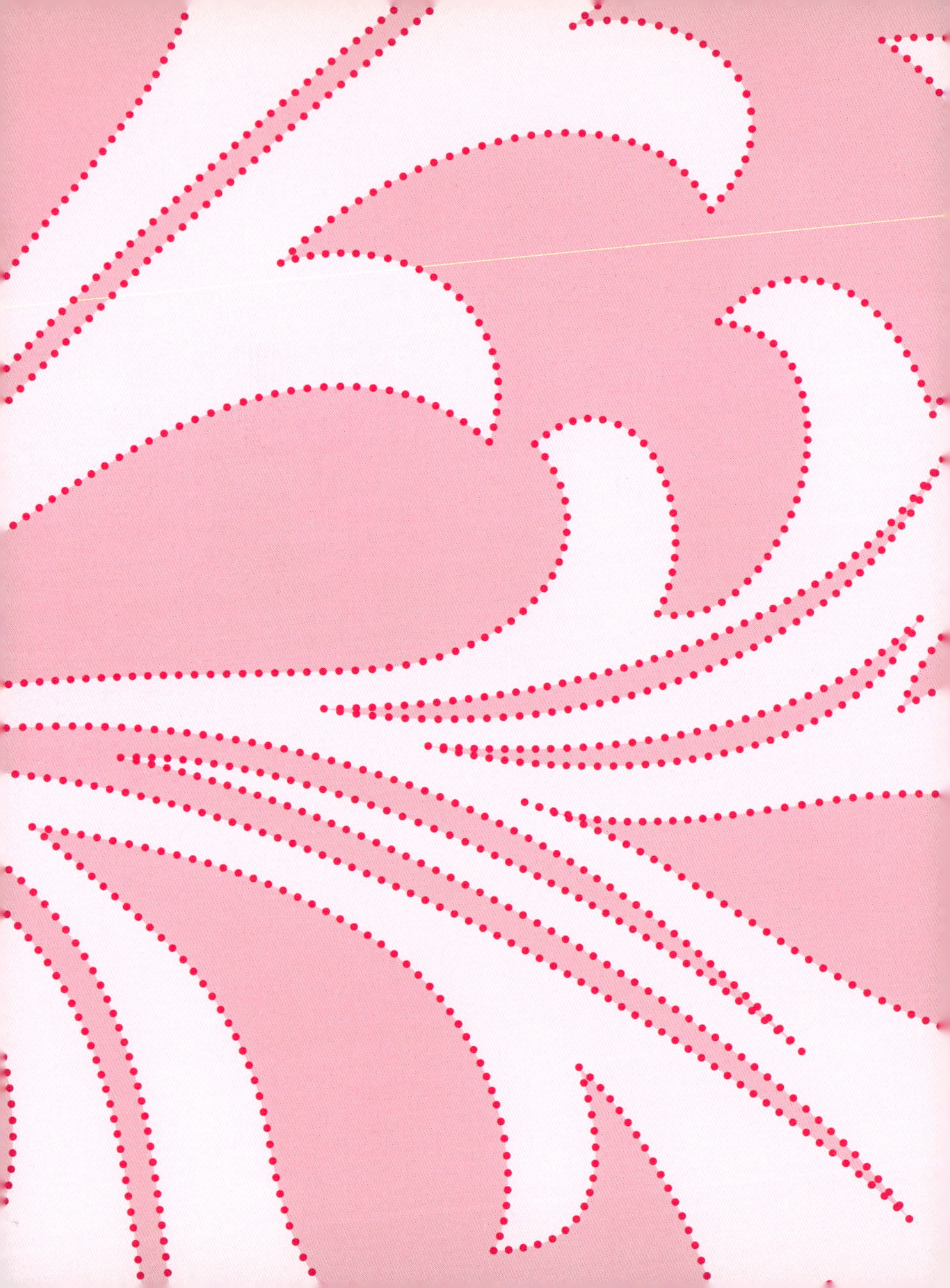

Chapter 6

Sexercise

Recipes for Lust

Your brain may be your most important sexual organ, but there's no getting around the fact that lovemaking gets better when the rest of your body is in shape. Studies on the relationship between sensational sex and health keep coming up with the same finding: just like keeping your car in tip-top condition, the key to a really good sex life (i.e., one that includes not just regular but teeth-rattling orgasms) is proper maintenance.

This isn't about transforming yourself into the female Schwarzenegger; it's about discovering and toning little-known muscles and hormones that contribute to more intense, enjoyable, even transcendent lovemaking for both of you.

The best news is, all it takes to improve your sex life forever is five short weeks. Think you have what it takes to enter the winner's circle? Then look no further for a get-fit plan that will keep you coming – and coming back for more.

Let the games begin!

★★★ GOLD You're in your oh! zone

★★ SILVER Feel the burn

★ BRONZE Heavy breathing

Hormone Heaven

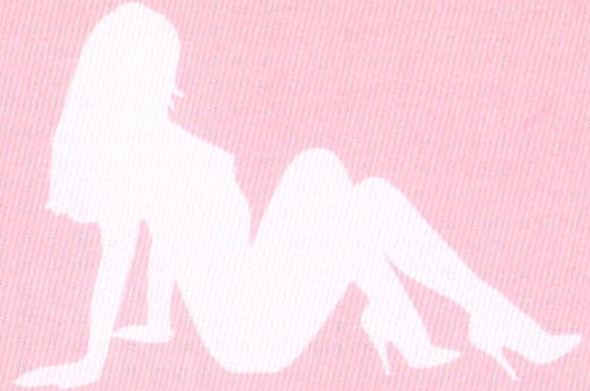

Getting a grip on your menstrual cycle will help you get the most out of it as a love machine.

Rejoice when your period comes. Science has found that those monthly changes in your levels of oestrogen and its sister hormones are what affect the intensity of your orgasms and give you a strong, flexible vagina, and regular production of cervical and vaginal lubricants.

Another happy by-product of following your hormonal peaks is that oestrogen and progesterone are defenders against STDs within your reproductive tract (although no one's suggesting this means you should skimp on the protection).

KEY DAYS FOR YOUR CALENDAR

The average length of a cycle is 28 days. Start counting from the first day of your period.

★ It's Day 10 and you feel marvellous, darling. Your oestrogen levels are at their pre-ovulatory peak and you are in the mood for love.

★ Know where your man is on Day 14. It's ovulation time which means testosterone (always present in your blood at a low level) spikes just as oestrogen crests, making you feel sexually aggressive. Your libido's raging and you're at your most man-magnetic. By the way, your body's also primed to get pregnant right now, so don't forget contraception!

★ Day 18 and you're in seductive mode – rising levels of oxytocin, the touch hormone, trigger a lust to touch and be touched. Now! BONUS: this hormone also sets off the uterine contractions that go with orgasm.

★ Make love on Day 28. Your brain misreads uterine puffiness as a sign of sexual arousal and actually craves orgasmic release. Wowza, wowza!

The Phwoargasm Diet

This no-deprivation diet will raise your ahhh-q.

★ Phosphorus has direct impact on sexual desire. Try food enriched with the miracle mineral (almonds, scallops, cheddar cheese, wheat bran, brewer's yeast and sunflower seeds) for glow-in-the-dark pleasure.

★ Honey pollen stimulates reproductive systems. Swallow the pollen in tablet form or stir granules straight into food.

★ According to nutritionists, cooking with garlic, ginger, pepper and onion helps perk up your libido by getting your blood pumping (but carry a breath mint for afterwards!).

★ Vegetarians might just be on to something. Researchers at the US Department of Agriculture have found that the mineral boron is vital for hormone production and sexual function. Boron can be found in dark green leafy vegetables, fruits (not citrus), nuts and legumes.

★ Take your vitamins. You need 45-plus nutrients daily to maintain good health (translation: regular orgasms). Even minor deficiencies can weaken the libido. Here's what you need to stockpile for better bliss.

Vitamin B (bread and yogurt) converts sugar and starches into energy, which translates into more stamina in bed.
Vitamin E (spinach, oatmeal, asparagus, eggs, nuts, brown rice, fruit), also known as the sex vitamin, is the one to pop to perk up passion.
Zinc (fish, oysters, liver, mushroom, grains, fresh fruit) increases testosterone levels in men and women. University of Rochester researchers found that men with zinc-deficient diets are at high risk of low libido and sex problems like infertility and prostrate problems (his pleasure-zone gland).
Vitamin D and calcium (milk, cheese) keep bones strong to do tricky positions without embarrassing fractures.

★ Go for a java jolt. A University of Michigan study found that compared to those who did not drink coffee, regular black oil drinkers were considerably more sexually active. WARNING: Caffeine can also deliver a performance-boosting jolt to sperm cells, increasing both their velocity (speed) and motility (liveliness).

★ Go ahead and eat that Cadbury's. Chocolate contains not only caffeine but also phenylethylamine (PEA), dubbed the 'molecule of love' by sexual medicine specialist Theresa Crenshaw, MD, author of The Alchemy of Love and Lust. A natural form of the stimulant amphetamine, a dose of PEA can increase lust levels to red-hot (the artificial sweetener aspartame also contains PEA so for those watching their weight, a Diet Coke will have the same effect).

Love Saboteurs

Not in the mood? Before blaming your partner, check out your medicine cabinet, diet, birth control and lifestyle.

PROBLEM: Fatigue.
SOLUTION: Use your bed … to sleep in, that is. Research shows that you need a minimum of 6 – 8 hours sleep a night to feel energized for lots of sex.

PROBLEM: Smoking.
SOLUTION: Kick ash. It seems that quitting the butt habit can make a bigger difference in your life than exercising. A study at the University of California at San Diego found that tobacco reduces testosterone levels and constricts blood flow, which has a less than smoking effect on your orgasms.

PROBLEM: Contraception.
SOLUTION: Take your Pill. A study at McGill University, Montreal, found that Pill users report more frequent and more satisfactory sex than non-users. Possible reasons: lighter menstrual periods, reduced PMS, mental security against pregnancy and the spontaneity of this method allows them to relax and enjoy the moment more.

PROBLEM: The Pill. It contains progesterone, a hormone that diminishes lubrication, sex drive and delays climax. You may still want sex and even enjoy it but the ultimate orgasmic blast-off can become a huge, labour-intensive effort. Hormonal implants can have the same effect.
SOLUTION: Switch to triphasic pills which have different levels of progesterone and, a San Francisco State University study found, may actually even increase desire.

PROBLEM: Your medicine prescription. Research by the Sex/Drug Interaction Foundation in California estimates that up to 20 per cent of all sex problems are caused by drug side effects or interactions. Certain asthma, blood-pressure, diabetes and migraine medications, synthetic androgens (used to treat endometriosis), heartburn soothers, antibiotics and beta blockers (used to treat cardiovascular disease) will all short-circuit desire and orgasm.
SOLUTION: Talk to your doctor about gentler alternative treatments.

PROBLEM: Over-the-counter sex stoppers. Antihistamines, decongestants and sleep aids are muscles relaxants – and you need muscle tension to reach orgasm. In addition, they can dry out the body's mucous membranes, making intercourse uncomfortable.
SOLUTION: Read the label before you buy. If it says, 'May cause drowsiness', it can also impair sexual desire or performance.

PROBLEM: Depression. Selective serotonin re-uptake inhibitors (SSRIs) – like Prozac, Zoloft and Paxil – have been found to have a downing effect on your sexuality, causing lowered libido, lack of arousal, delay in orgasm or reduction in orgasmic intensity.
SOLUTION: A lower dose might reduce sexual side effects while preserving antidepressant effects. Or try a drug holiday (check with your doctor first). A study by MacLean Hospital in Massachusetts found that more than half of those taking antidepressants reported better sexual functioning and more desire when they had drug-free weekends (Thursday noon to Sunday noon).

PROBLEM: Booze. Ironically, we drink to lower inhibition. But alcohol also lowers sex drive. A general rule of thumb is that the amount of alcohol it takes to affect your driving (for an average-size woman, one to two drinks an hour) will also affect your libido.
SOLUTION: Get your high naturally with exercise.

PROBLEM: Your diet. Big pre-thang meals can affect you in much the same way as alcohol. It makes you feel fat, sleepy, and you sweat what you eat. Lovely!
SOLUTION: Lighten up on the heavy meals, especially those containing fatty oils and butter. See page 158–9 for ingredients that'll keep you purring with pleasure.

PROBLEM: His knickers. Besides studies showing that tight briefs might affect his sperm count, lower back moves while wearing tight gym shorts can result in a painful swelling known as stretcher's scrotum.
SOLUTION: Make sure he hangs loose at all times.

PROBLEM: He's a cyclist. Too much wheeling can result in Alcock Syndrome (numb willy from too much bicycle riding).
SOLUTION: Help him get his exercise in other ways (like lying down).

The Love Workout

Ever tried a new position, only to find that while the mind is willing, the thighs are screaming, 'How long do you expect me to keep this up?' Unlike most full-contact sports, you can't call time-out during lovemaking. Which is why trimming the flab, toning muscles and building stamina are vital to getting good sex (good hygiene and ace blow job skills don't hurt either). An orgasm is essentially a series of contractions of the uterine, vaginal, rectal and pubococcygeus (PC) muscles. Ergo, the stronger your muscles, the stronger the contractions, the more pleasure you'll feel and the more control you'll have over your own – and your lover's – bliss.

All it takes is 20 minutes of exercise a week to develop killer love muscles. Keep it moderate (around 145 heartbeats per minute) or you'll be too whacked to get whacked. Expect results within weeks.

One word of caution all you A-type personalities: take it easy. In the sex/exercise connection, more isn't better (good news). Too much muscle soreness and fatigue can easily put a damper on romance while over-rigorous training can cause hormonal imbalances in your libido. Three times a week is more than enough to feel results.

Just Do It

It's official: A hard body leads to better whoa! It starts with the heart. In a study of nearly 3,000 men and women by the University of California at San Diego, it was found that as fitness levels improve, so does cardiovascular endurance. This means a greater volume of blood can be pumped throughout the body – genitals included. And blood circulation is key for a man's erection and a woman's arousal system (it increases lubrication and clitoral swelling).

★ Don't be afraid to break a sweat – perspiration is actually an aphrodisiac packed with come-hither-and-ravage-me pheromones (up the stakes by chucking away your deodorant). In Shakespeare's time, a woman hoping to attract a man tucked a peeled apple in her armpit and then offered this 'love apple' to the object of her lust.

★ Another reason to skip your post-workout shower and steam up in bed instead: exercise also stimulates the endocrine glands, making testosterone levels in both men and women rise sharply. Translation: you want it and you want it now.

★ If you're healthy and in good shape, you may climax more easily. Sex therapist Dr Linda De Villers studied more than 8,000 women and found regular exercisers had more intense and fulfilling orgasms – perhaps because people who workout take pride in their bodies and have higher self-esteem. (It's harder to have an orgasm if you're obsessing over the size of your bum.)

★ Stay motivated with this news: A study at the University of Texas in Austin found that working out makes you horny. When you exercise, heart rate and blood pressure are elevated and the blood vessels in the genitals become primed for action. Result: post-workout sex is bound to be explosive.

★ Finally, exercise keeps nerves in tip-top shape, sharpening the ability to feel and focus on all bodily sensations (and tune out that annoying 'Did I pay the electricity bill?' voice). Continue toning exercises during your lovemaking for the ultimate sensual experience!

★ Don't leave him on the couch. After nine months of working out for one hour three times a week, your man is likely to have a shorter post-ejaculation recovery period. Hello, orgasmic hat tricks!

★ The American Council on Exercise reports that burning at least 200 calories a day exercising (the equivalent of walking two miles briskly) can keep his willy perky and interested, preventing or even reversing premature ejaculation, low libido and penile droop.

Sweat It Out

Key cardio moves for getting hot and bothered.

- ★ Alternate your aerobic days with a weight-training regimen that covers the full body – arms, legs, abdomen, chest and back. Use either free weights or a weight machine system like Nautilus. The goal is to increase strength and tone muscles, so work with a weight that's about half of what you're capable of lifting. Do three sets of 12 repetitions for each muscle group. ★★

- ★ Start pounding the pavement. In one poll, 66 per cent of the men and women runners interviewed claimed that regular jogging made them better lovers. Alternatively, put a spin on your workouts; in another poll, two-thirds of cycling enthusiasts said the exercise made them better lovers. ★★

- ★ Lap it up for long-lasting juiciness. A Harvard University study of middle-aged swimmers concluded that men and women over 40 who got wet regularly were as sexually active as people in their late twenties and early thirties. And they enjoyed it more. ★★

- ★ For explosive results, go from almost no exercise to three one-hour workouts a week. One study found that this technique results in a 30 per cent increase in how often you play the field, a 20 per cent increase in tonsil hockey and a decrease in being benched because of non-working parts. ★★★

TIP: You don't have to schedule a gym trip every time you want to have sex. The kind of breathlessness necessary for a precoital charge can also be had from a rowdy, bawdy pillow fight with your lover. Tickling, wrestling and fighting can all also set off sparks. ★

Pelvis Power

Forget upper arms as taut as cables and a bum so firm you can flip a coin off of it – the stronger your and his pelvic muscles are, the tighter you'll be able to contract during sex and squeeze out every last drop of pleasure.

LIBIDO LIFTER: Lie flat with your arms at your sides, knees bent and feet flat on the floor. Raise your hips as high as you can and hold for a count of three, then lower them until your body nearly touches the floor. Do triple sets of ten three times a week for pumping endurance that a WWF wrestler would envy. ★★

THE THRUST: A variation of the Libido Lifter, above. Lie down as before, then raise your hips so your bum is the only part of your body off the floor. Slowly rock or tilt your pelvis up while exhaling and down while inhaling. Repeat slowly and smoothly 20 times. ★★

THE TILT: Open the muscles of the pelvic floor by getting down on all fours with your hands directly beneath your shoulders and your knees under your hips. On a long, slow inhalation, lower your belly and lift your pelvis, then look towards the ceiling. On the exhalation, arch your back upwards, drop your head and tuck your tailbone forward. Slowly and smoothly alternate between these poses for about 30 seconds, focusing on the movement in your pelvis. ★★

ROCK-AND-ROLL: Stand and swivel your hips, doing a rolling motion as if you're doing a bad Elvis imitation. Move only your hips, not your shoulders or upper body. Do this for one or two minutes at various speeds once or twice a day. ★

Lift It

Before you do the limbo of love, beef up with these never-gruelling-always-gratifying strength-training moves that target your erotic core.

SHOULDERS: To keep you in shape for staying on top (which is, incidentally, the best position to stimulate the G-spot and other sensitive areas in the vagina, such as its end).
WORK IT: Sit up. Hold your arms above your head and cross your wrists. Inhale, straightening your arms. Extend them back behind your head as far as possible, keeping your wrists crossed (your elbows should be behind your ears). Hold for ten seconds, then relax. Repeat three times. ★★

UPPER ARMS: Strengthening the triceps will help you hold yourself up longer when you're on top.
WORK IT: Sit on a chair with its back against a wall, holding the front of the seat with the heels of your hands. Slide off the chair and freeze, with your knees bent, elbows facing the wall and arms supporting your body. Lower your body, bending your elbows to a 90-degree angle, then push up. Do three sets of 15. ★

ABDOMINALS: These are your orgasmic power centre. They help maintain your position, push your inner clitoris into the path of his penis, keep the lower back strong (important for those sexy thrusts) and hold your belly in (important when it comes to luring a partner to willingly do the aforementioned thrusting motions with you).
WORK IT: Sit up straight. Pull your belly button in for one second, imagining it's touching the back of your spine. Release. Repeat 99 times, counting aloud (so you don't hold your breath). Aim for five sets of 100 a day.
MIX IT IN: Squeeze your abs during sex – you'll beef up your orgasms to twice their usual size. ★★★

DERRIÈRE: Strengthening these muscles helps build pressure in your pelvic region.
WORK IT: Flex and release your bum rhythmically for about 20 seconds every day.
MIX IT IN: Clenching your buns together every couple of seconds during sex will push you both over the Big O brink. ★★★

BACK: Sex feels better than busting concrete, but your back muscles don't know the difference. Sex-related backaches are especially common when nearing climax, the point of maximum muscle tension.
WORK IT: Lie on your back and slowly bring your knees to your chest. Grab your knees and hold them against your chest for a few breaths, relaxing throughout the movement.
MIX IT IN: Elevate your legs by lying flat on the floor and propping your feet on the backs of his thighs during sex. This will take the pressure off the sciatic nerve and relax those hot twinges of a minor backache. ★

HIPS: Don't forget to hit below the belt. As the key pivot in the thrusting motion, your hip joints and muscles must remain flexible.
WORK IT: Push both thighs outwards and hold for thirty seconds. Relax. Repeat ten times.
MIX IT IN: Get on top – it's an instant hip easer. ★★★

INNER THIGHS: Necessary for those tricky standing-on-one-leg-on-a-tree moves.
WORK IT: Sit on a chair and squeeze your knees, pushing them together for about ten seconds. Repeat ten times, three times a day.
MIX IT IN: Do the squeeze during the missionary position – you'll create friction on the outer part of the clitoris and the inner folds of the vulva – yum! ★★

UPPER THIGHS: The quads – the muscles at the front of the thighs – are key players in any on-top position.
WORK IT: Stand 30 cm (1 ft) away from a wall, facing out. Lean back so your torso touches the wall. Slide down, bending your knees until your thighs are parallel to the floor. Hold for 30 seconds, building up to two minutes. ★

CALVES: This move stops you from overflexing your calf muscles during orgasm (and ending up with the wrong kind of spasms).
WORK IT: Lie flat on your back with one leg bent and one leg straight. Raise the straight leg as far as you can until it's pointing at the ceiling. Hold and exhale while slowly flexing your foot, pointing the toes down towards your chest. Relax, then lower the leg. Repeat three times on each leg.
MIX IT IN: Lock your legs around his hips and squeeze your calves, drawing him closer. ★★★

The Joy of Flex

It's not enough to be strong. You also want to be limber and loose. Studies have found that muscle tightness dramatically blocks the range of motion of the legs, hips and pelvis – all key players in sexual activity. In addition, most of us clench our muscles when aroused, trying to almost push ourselves into coming.

On the flip side, stretching pumps a lot of blood into muscles and that stimulates the nerves that run through them. And when you can relax and go slack and submit to ecstasy, your orgasm will simply come to you.

These stretches and breathing exercises will help you loosen up for every tight spot you want to get in. Designed to stretch and tone AND make you both moan, these should be done two or three times weekly to stay permanently loose or within several hours of a planned rendezvous to help you soar to a more aware and prolonged state of arousal.

Get a Buzz On

Breathe your way to erotic bliss.

★ To make it through the long haul, long-distance runners must learn to master their breathing. And if you want to make medal-winning moves on your mattress, you should do the same. Breathe deeply through your mouth, all the way down to your diaphragm. Once you have a rhythm going, speed it up breath by breath to raise the level of sexual excitement and push you over the finishing line.

★ Learn the seven chakra breaths. Inhale deeply so that your lower belly expands. Exhale slowly and fully, using the abdominal muscles to expel all of the air from the lungs. With each complete breath (inhale plus exhale), focus on the base of your spine (strength), uterus (sexuality), stomach (emotions), heart (love), throat (expression), forehead (intuition), and crown (individuality). This will open up all the places where there's tension, enhancing sensitivity, allowing pleasure in, heightening perception and increasing stamina. Make love immediately after doing this – it's more likely you'll have a whole body orgasm.

★ This only works when you know you're about to get lucky. Plug your left nostril for 15 minutes prior to the action starting and you'll increase the air flow to the sexier side of the brain, which really gets you in the mood. Of course, that tissue dangling from your nose might kill it.

★ Share a Tantric kiss: Sit on his lap. Inhale while he's exhaling. As he breathes out, suck his breath into your body, down to your sex organs. After one minute, kiss and share your breath. Intercourse may not even be necessary when you're so merged.

Stretch Yourself Sexy

Prepare for passion with these lusty moves to improve your let-me-at-him lunges.

★ Imagine the positions you want to get in for lovemaking and do them as stretches. Hold the pose, breathing deeply and stretching just a little more with each exhale. ★★

★ The psoas muscle is central for rocking the pelvis forward and back and side to side – moves that turn sex into an ooh-la-la experience. Strengthen yours with this yoga stretch. Stand with your knees slightly bent and inhale while gently rocking your pelvis back. Exhale as you smoothly return to your original position. Your weight should remain evenly balanced on your feet. ★★★

★ Shake your booty. During conventional orgasms, muscles get so charged and tense that they need release, and the experience is over. Standing and shaking out your body for 10 minutes, part by part, will let out tension and get energy flowing throughout your entire body, getting you ready for tip 95. ★★★

★ Release your inner groin muscles and shake hands with deeper, more fulfilling orgasms. Sit with your legs wide apart. Bring the soles of your feet together, resting on the outside of each foot. Draw your feet towards your pelvis and gently press their soles together to increase the stretch. Hold and breathe for one to two minutes. ★

★ Kneel with your bottom on your feet. Lean forward, resting your torso on the top of your thighs and stretching your arms out in front of you to loosen the muscles along your spine. Have your partner stand directly behind you and gently press your back to enhance the stretch. Switch places and repeat. This will loosen your upper, middle and lower back, making it easier to have an orgasmic triathlon. ★★

★ Get a quick lift when you feel drained by lowering your head, flipping your hair forward and pressing on the back of your head. This area is your energy zone and stretching it boosts circulation (the secret to all good orgasms). Extra pick-you-up-and-push-you-over-the-edge tip: spritz the area with a sharp, spicy fragrance containing musk or ylang ylang. ★

★ Knead out those knots. A sensual massage will turn up the body heat in more ways than one. Athletes get massages to increase circulation to the muscle groups. The increased blood flow warms the muscles so they'll stretch more easily and perform to their fullest capacity. To ensure personal-best sexual performance, dab a few drops of massage oil or lotion on your hands and place them, palms flat, on your partner's lower back. Run your palms in small circles up his back, along both sides of his spine, all the way up to his shoulders. Have him do the same for you. ★★

Get Spiritual

Shape up with this no-sweat Tantric workout.

1. Connect: dim the lights, then sit facing each other, gazing into each other's eyes for at least five minutes.

2. Lay head-to-head on the floor so that your bodies form one long line. Nestle your heads on each other's shoulders. The goal is to relax and tune into each other until you can breathe together – it'll take about ten minutes.

3. Sit facing each other and redo step 1.

4. Place your hands on each other's chests, feeling both your hearts beat. Breathe (see Get a Buzz On, page 168–9).

5. Kiss. Taste each other everywhere. When you become really excited, stop and return to step 1. It's important not to work up too much of a sweat – Tantric-style sex is calm and restful. Keep your head clear while your body gets turned on.

6. Almost do it, position 1: Get into your O-Zone – get on top with your body resting on his chest and your shins flat on the mattress. He enters you partially – an inch every five minutes (don't measure!). Lay still as long as you can. Do your Kegels (see page 172) to help him stay erect. When you can't take it any more, start stroking and kissing, but stop after 20 minutes, letting your bodies go limp so you don't come.

7. Almost do it, position 2: He lays on his side while you lay on your back with your legs over his and your bodies at a 45-degree angle and continue as step 6.

8. Now really do it, position 3: Repeat steps 1 to 4. Then sit on his lap so that you're facing him. This time, let yourself go completely for a total gut-busting orgasm that will stay with you for days.

The Intercourse Orgasm

Time to use the greatest piece of fitness equipment ever invented: a bed.

Anyone who's limber, toned and in shape can make love like a rabbit. But sex is more like synchronized swimming than a 100-metre dash. Timing, in other words, is everything. Bottom line: a strong tongue muscle is only going to get you so far between the sheets. What you need to do is add some exercises and stretches that target the parts of the body called into play during lovemaking, giving you more control over and more intensity during your orgasm. These following high-voltage moves will help boost your performance and give your sex life more pleasure than a lifetime supply of sex toys.

Pump It Up

Studies have found that stronger pubococcygeus (PC) muscles make women more orgasmic more frequently and men more likely to experience multiple orgasms. Here's your four-step guide to gold-standard love muscles.

1 The easiest way to locate your PCs is to try to stop your urine flow mid-stream (don't do this more than once a day, as it may irritate your bladder).

2 Once you have a general idea of where your PC is, practise the basic Kegel exercise. You can do this in any position, but you'll probably find it most comfortable to do while sitting in a chair or lying on your back. Squeeze your PC, hold for three seconds, then release. Repeat until you can build up to 100 at a time.

3 According to Dr Cynthia Mervis Watson, co-author of *Love Potions: A Doctor's Guide to Aphrodisia*, the exercise should be done with your legs slightly apart

rather than with your thighs clamped together. You will find that you are drawing your pelvis upwards, but if you find the exercise tiring, it may be that you're also tensing your buttocks and abdomen; try to isolate only your PC muscles.

4 Place a hand on your abdomen while contracting to ensure that it's relaxed. Inserting a finger into your vagina or placing a hand at the opening also helps identify the movement and confirm that you're squeezing the right muscles.

★ Now use your pumped-up muscles to milk him to orgasm. During sex, move your hips very slowly up and down his penis' shaft while squeezing your PCs so you can apply varying amounts of pressure to his organ. Mix in the pelvic moves in Rock-and-Roll on page 165 to get his penis to give you a massage at the same time. ★★

★ Crush him. When you're a groan away from climax, let loose by rapidly fluttering your PC muscles – squeezing faster with shorter pauses in between. Flex five times quickly. The harder and more rapidly you squeeze, the stronger your and his orgasm will be. ★★★

★ Boogie slow and easy. Powerfully squeeze your PCs in a constricting manner to push him out. Repeat on the in-stroke, this time squeezing to pull him back in. Push out, constrict, pull in a little and push out and constrict again. When you've developed enough strength, you should be able to keep it up all night. ★

★ Twist to the corkscrew: With your knees bent, lie on top of your partner, who is on his back with his penis inside you. Resting on his chest, squeeze his penis and slowly circle your hips five times. Stop and release the squeeze. Then squeeze hard again and rotate your hips in the other direction. Continue the cycle until you are both ready to pop. ★

★ Get him to prod your hot spots. During sex, push down with your PCs to bring the front wall of your vagina down to meet his penis. This helps him tickle your G-spot. (Combine this with the Tilt on page 165 to make this a Gold.) ★★★

Let's Get Physical

Research has found that the couple who sweat together also sizzle together – they have sex more often and more orgasms when they do it. For an added incentive, do the sexercises naked.

★ Push-ups tone the chest and arms, making it a cinch to get on top (not to mention fuelling chandelier-swinging abilities). Kneel and place your palms in his hands. Slowly lower and push back up (kisses on the down move make a good incentive). Repeat ten times. ★★

★ Do the body tug to strengthen your inner thighs, lower back, arms and abs. Sit facing your partner, keeping your backs straight and tall. With his legs straight and spread in a wide V, extend your thighs and place your feet along his inner thighs. Reach your arms across to one another, clasp hands and look directly into each other's eyes. Maintaining eye contact, lean back as far as you can while he leans in towards you. Take turns leaning forwards and back. Switch inside and outside legs and repeat. ★★★

★ Do a high-five for a whole-body workout. Stand very close to your partner, face to face. Both of you bend down into a squat, then jump up as high as you can and slap hands (and any other body parts you care to connect) together. ★

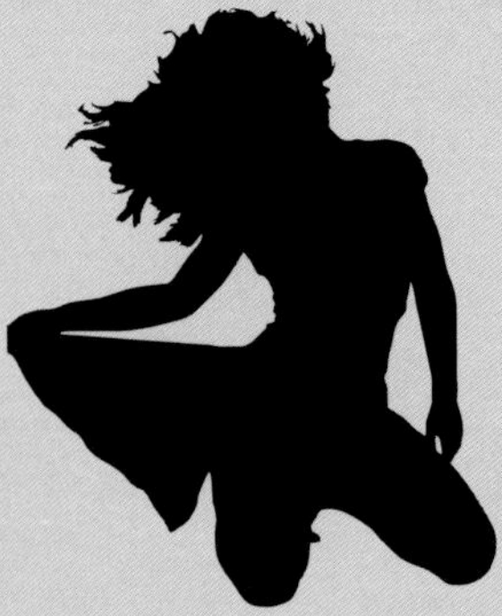

★ Do a better crunch. Instead of the abs workout on page 166, place your feet high on his chest (to prevent your back from arching) and contract your stomach, bringing your shoulders closer to your knees. Do two sets of 25 repetitions each. ★★

★ The pelvic tilt will keep hips, abs and thighs granite hard. Combine this with squeezing your PCs and you'll be a sex engine. Lie on your back with your knees bent and your feet flat on the floor. Rest your arms by your sides and have your partner kneel beside you. As you raise your pelvis slowly off the floor, have him place his hands under you to help you hold the posture, making sure your hips and thighs are in line. Lower your pelvis to the floor and repeat. ★★★

★ To strengthen the lower back, hang your upper body off the bed while he sits on your thighs to stabilize you. Then raise your torso just past horizontal, hold for one beat and lower. Repeat eight times. ★★

★ Place your feet high on his chest, supporting his body weight. Slowly lower him, bringing your knees to your chest. Push him back to the starting position (penetration is optional). Repeat five times. ★★★

★ Let him be your stretching rack. Sit with your legs apart, his feet above your ankles. As you relax forward, he gently pulls your arms to deepen the stretch (repeat twice). ★

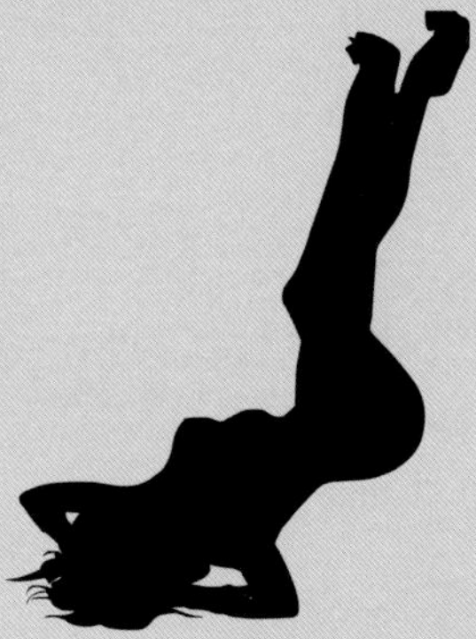

Passion Pole Vaults

These moves count not only as great sex, but also great exercise. Get ready to do victory laps. * For these exercises you can easily switch places so he gets the workout as well.

PRESS DOWN*

TARGETS: Shoulders.

DO IT: Have your partner lie face up underneath you. He penetrates, then moves up and down by doing push-ups that are about half the range of movement of standard ones. ★

PUSH BACK

TARGETS: Triceps.

DO IT: Start from a sitting position on the floor. Lean back, supporting your weight with your hands behind you and your fingers pointing forward. Have your partner slip between your thighs with his knees and hands on the floor, his head just over your shoulder. Pick your bum off the ground. Once he lowers himself onto (and into) you, you do the work. From a bent-elbow starting position, thrust towards him by straightening your arms. Bend again. For more sextension, he can lean against you until you're supporting most of his weight. ★★

LOVE CURL*

TARGETS: Biceps.

DO IT: Stand about 90 cm (3 ft) away from the wall, with your back to it. Lean your lower back and shoulders against the wall. He should lie on you with his chest to yours, his legs pressed against you and his penis inside you. Scoop your arms around him so your hands are resting against his shoulder blades. He leans back until your arms are extended (take care he doesn't slip out). Slowly curl him back to you. To make it easier, he can put his arms around you and help pull himself up. ★

SQUATTER*

TARGETS: Quads and hamstrings.

DO IT: Have him squat low, leaning back against a wall. Squat over him, making sure you keep your knees bent at a right angle. Move up and down on his penis by pressing with your thighs (if this is too hard, you can give him some of your weight by putting your hands on his thighs). ★★★

BODY BEND

TARGETS: Upper back.

DO IT: Stand with your back to him and your knees bent, leaning slightly forward. Plant your legs firmly with your feet 45 cm (18 in) apart. Have him drape himself over you and penetrate you from behind. Placing your hands on your thighs, support his weight, using your upper back to move you both up and down. ★

Work It

Slip these drills into your regular sex routine and he'll be bending over backwards to please you.

★ Break orgasm time records. During oral sex or intercourse, have your man support you by slipping his hands under your hips and lifting your pelvis up while you clench your bum muscles.

★ Put pressure on your abs. Your lower abdomen, just above the pubic hairline, is basically the outside of the inner clitoris. Squeezing the ab muscles intensifies the feeling inside. Do a mini sit-up during sex to tip you over the edge, as it will sandwich your inner clitoris between two hard surfaces (i.e., your tensed muscles and his penis).

★ Open and close your legs in small pumps during sex. Doing this will trigger orgasm in two ways: first, closing your legs makes it easier to clench those thigh muscles, which actually continue far enough to stimulate your inner clitoris. Second, opening and closing creates friction on the outer visible part of the clitoris and the inner folds of the vulva.

An Orgasm a Day

Newsflash: There is a pain-free way to boost looks, improve health, lower stress, make periods pain-free, reduce stress, lift moods, increase confidence and keep you in peak condition.

What is this unknown road to fabulousness?

Sex. And lots of it.

OK, so you may not wake up with perfectly highlighted tresses, Brad Pitt and a fantastic TV sitcom contract. But it turns out that orgasms don't just feel good. They're also good for you. Because sexual arousal and orgasm involve the interplay of several body systems, it's now known that even a common-or-garden-variety shag does more for your physical wellbeing than a month-long holiday in Tahiti.

These are all the glorious reasons why getting physical will make you look and feel more beautiful (as if you needed an excuse to have more sex!).

The Look of Love

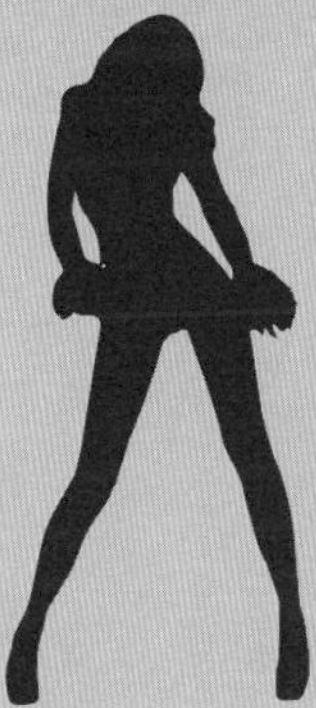

Making love is a painless way to make you look better (and much cheaper than visiting a spa!). Here's how.

★ Who needs collagen when you have regular sex? A single make-out session can act as a luscious lip-puffer-upper that would make even Angelina Jolie bite her lips.

★ A snog a day keeps the cosmetic surgeon away. Kissing has been recognized as one of the best facial exercises around. Experts say that all that puckering tones up facial muscles, keeping you looking young and beautiful.

★ The only cover-up you need for your skin is a sexy little number. When Mr Desirable touches you, you get such an explosive rush that it sends blood rushing to the surface, making your heart beat faster and blood pressure rise. It's this rollercoaster of love that makes you positively glow after sex.

★ Toss away those AHA creams. According to an Ohio University study, orgasm increases your lymphocyte numbers (the cells responsible for fighting physical degeneration) – so regular climaxes could make you remain gorgeous well into old age.

★ Here's an inexpensive conditioner – sex is known to stimulate the hormones which give your hair a healthy, shiny sheen.

★ A little bit of sex can help you get away with shaving a few years off your age. A Royal Edinburgh Hospital in Scotland study found that sex helps you look between four and seven years younger because it helps you feel more content, sleep better and feel less stressed.

★ Regular lovemaking increases a woman's oestrogen level, which keeps the skin and vaginal tissues supple, moist and glowing.

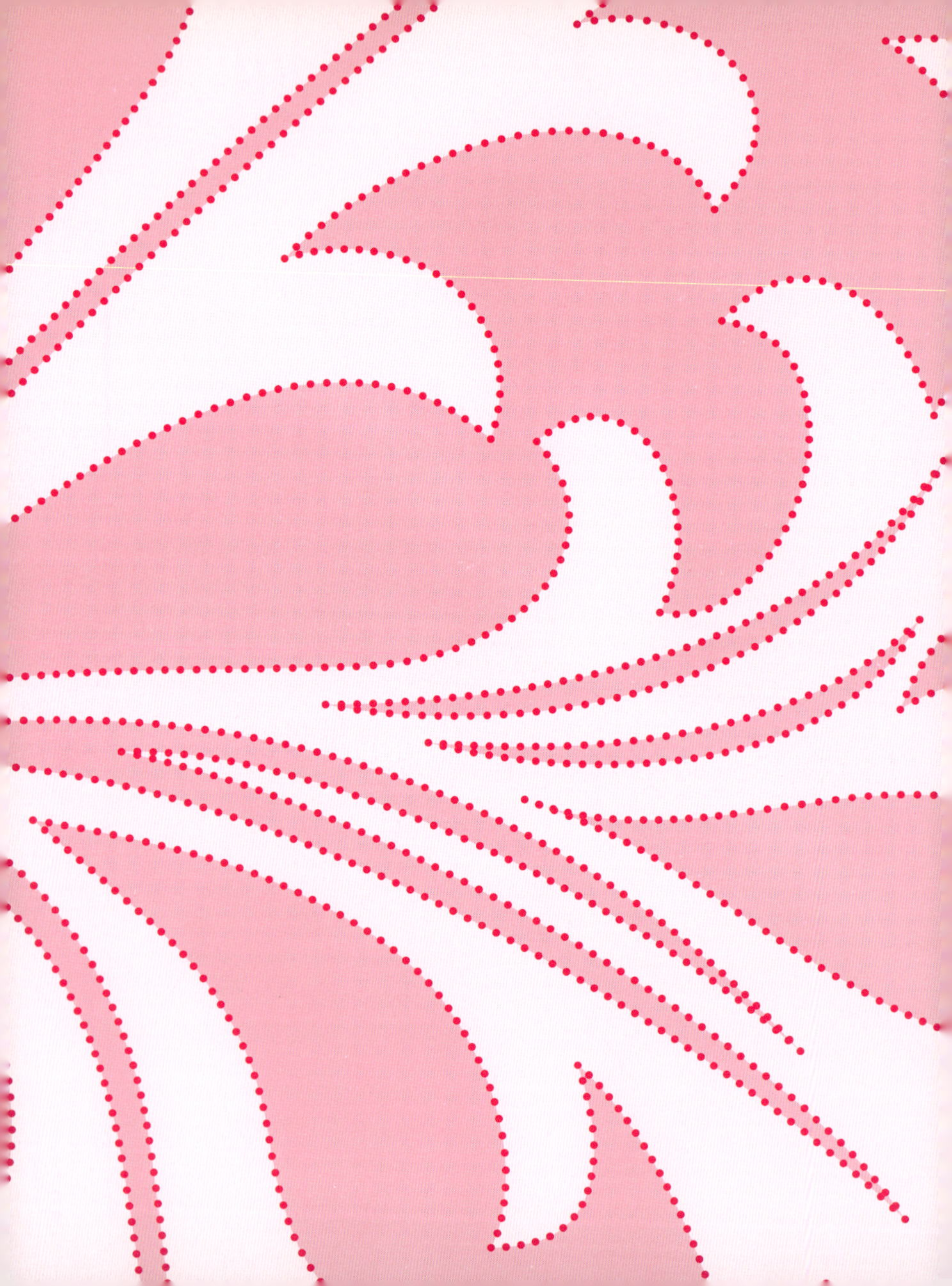

Chapter 7

Triple X Sex Tricks

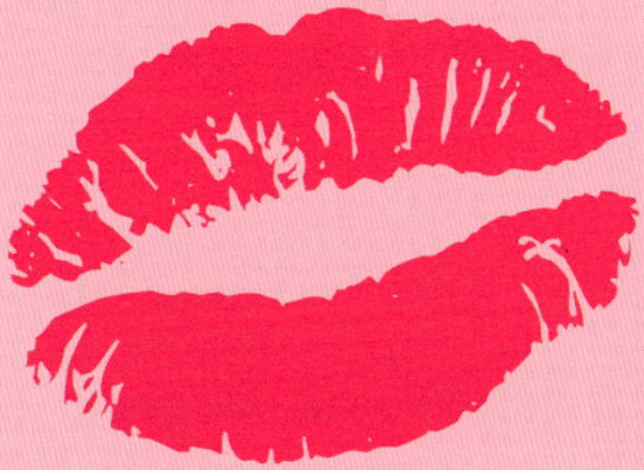

THRILL LEVEL

When appropriate, text is rated to determine the Triple X level as follows:

S: Steam it up

E: Edgy and Wild

X: Extreme Kink

Max Out Your Pleasure

Even good sex can become routine. The good news is that it's easy to add a jolt to routine sex. Just take a stroll on the wild side.

Doing something you've never done before can send your system into overdrive. When you go beyond your limits, you discover hidden turn-ons and new sensations – maybe even a hot zone you never knew you had. Plus, your willingness to explore your sexual boundaries will help build intimacy and trust between you and your partner. When you think about it … is there any reason *not* to have a naughty day?

Pillow Talk

Truly amazing erotic action can happen only when both partners are willing to take risks. Here are eight steps to calm your lover's fears and to get them involved in your secret desires (and liking it!) without setting off perv alarms.

1 Don't beg. Don't grovel. It's not seemly. And it's not necessary. Your best move is to give the relationship a month or two before breaking out the vibe.

2 Make sure they know they can melt you down sans kink.

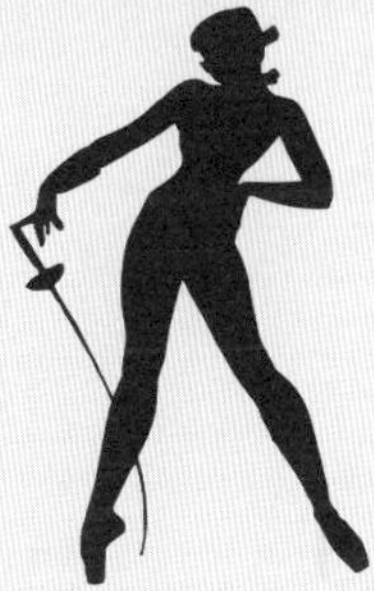

3 A weekend away is a good time to get the ball rolling. A change of scenery makes people more open to new things.

4 When the time comes, don't jump right in and unload. Here are a few strategies for talking yourself into a wilder sex life.

* If you're shy: Don't bother talking. Instead, slyly test the waters – see how they react to doing something slightly off from your usual routine. Get into a new position or hold their wrists down. If they act unruffled, they're probably open to listening to the idea of doing something a bit unusual. **S**
* If you're bold: Ask about the best sex they've ever had. Or their favourite fantasy. Discovering what they like instead of barking out your wants will make your partner feel less intimidated. Hopefully, they will start asking what you like, too. After you tell them, you can show them. **E**
* If you're a risk taker: Offer to be their sex slave for the entire day. **X**

5 Simplify by using a visual aid. You can get a video or book with a scene that illustrates your deepest desire. The key, though, is to be specific – 'Do you see that? That makes me really hot.' **S**

6 Take a leaf from the Kama Sutra. Breaching carnal taboos doesn't sound freaky when it reads like poetry. Instead of asking your lover if they want to try it up the bum, ask if they'd enjoy 'flower congress'. Doesn't that sound much better? **S**

7 Be prepared for the need for some damage control. If you went too far, too fast, here's some phrases to memorize to keep them from running into the night.

* Sorry, you just looked so hot lying/bending/bouncing like that, I couldn't resist.
* I've never had anyone do that with me before, and I wanted to know what it would be like. You're the first person I've felt comfortable enough to ask.
* Just kidding!

8 Quit while you're ahead. If they flinched when you climbed on top, it's probably not a great idea to break out the fuzzy cuffs.

Rules of the Game

Erotic extras spice up the bedroom, but they can also backfire. Beware of these passion poopers (all players must read the following before starting).

- ★ Heating it up: Nuking marshmallows, chocolate sauce or honey and dripping it over each other's body sounds like a sweet idea, but the results can actually be too hot for lovers and cause surface skin burns (same goes for candle wax). Stay in lukewarm territory (if you can dip your finger in without agony, it's probably OK).

- ★ Beware alien invasions: Don't use any object that's not specifically designed for that part of the body – inserting certain fruit and veggies (see next tip for the exceptions), cooking tools and candles in the vagina for instance. But also anal vibrators in the vagina, rubber bands around the penis and so on. You can cause an irritation at the very least and serious injury in a worst-case scenario (do you really want to explain how the vacuum cleaner nozzle got stuck up your bottom?).

- ★ Eat your fruit and vegetables: As long as you don't use any food that can break off or get stuck in the vaginal canal, inserting food is no more dangerous than inserting a dildo. Things that potentially will not come out are off limits (like grapes). Avoid spicy foods because they could burn. If you use sweet foods near your vaginal area, wash well afterwards to prevent yeast infections. Anything with oil in it (such as chocolate or whipped cream) can burn holes in latex birth control.

- ★ Check what's in your lube. Some aren't safe to use with latex, others will harm silicone toys.

- ★ Don't be a blow-hard: If air is blown directly into the vagina during oral sex, there's a risk it'll accidentally create an air embolus – an air bubble that blocks the passage of blood in an artery or vein – which could have lethal consequences.

- ★ Say what you mean and mean what you say. If you tell your lover, 'I just want to tie up your hands' and as soon as they oblige, you fasten their feet too, they'll never play cops and robbers with you again – you messed with their trust.

★ Before starting, make sure you're packing the right tools. Like if they've agreed to let you go knockin' at the back door, have lube ready and waiting. Or if you're filming your action, make sure the camera is charged up.

★ Only the brave (and probably not too bright) would let a partner render them helpless after a few dates. Know your partner before getting tied up. And never divulge personal info to a cyber-buddy.

★ Before trying anything new, make a code word to stop play. This way, if your lover does something too freaky, you can alert them – immediately. Especially if you're all tied up. Make it an attention-grabber like 'Vinegar'. 'Stop' doesn't work because they may think it's of the 'Stop, it feels so good' variety, as opposed to 'I want everything to stop NOW, no more games, scene over, let me outta here!'

★ Ignore pain at your peril. Sure, sometimes getting kinky is about upping the fear factor. But if that clamp is turning their extremities blue, don't ruin the moment by forcing them to go on. If spanking is part of your play, keep away from kidneys, liver, spleen or tailbone.

★ When tying things up, keep it loose – circulation is a good thing, especially in all the right parts. Tight scarves and handcuffs can cause numbness; blocking the nose or mouth can make you hyperventilate or induce a panic attack. And never tie anything around the neck. It's also good to have scissors on hand in case Mother shows up unannounced.

★ Everyone likes sex, but you should never be willing to die for it. HIV and AIDS are more easily spread through anal sex than any other sexual act, so always wear a condom when entering through the back door. Another rule of the rear is never to let him double-dip from bottom to vagina without re-rubbering up.

★ Wash all toys according to manufacturer's recommendations – it'll extend the life of your playthings as well as keep you infection-free.

Bust Out of Your Sex Rut

Five really easy things to get you started on the path to the wild side – and no, you won't need any special equipment. These all have a guaranteed **S** rating.

1 Buy some PVC, leather or suede. Start small with a glove or a bit of material that you can lie on, wear or rub between your legs or anywhere else that takes your fancy when you make love.

2 Hardcore players use slings purposely designed for some wild fun but you can get the same sensation with a cheap hammock. Hang it in a corner of your lounge so it looks like an innocent design feature. Then get down and dirty when the lights are out. **TIP:** Lying-down hammock sex will just make you feel seasick. Instead, he should stand on the edge while you do position gymnastics.

3 Wrap a silk scarf around your hand. Rubit all over your lover's body, especially back and forth between the thighs and against the crotch. Tie it around his nuts and bolts, then tie a large knot with about 30 cm (12 in) of fabric on either end to hold onto. As you ride him, pull on the free ends so that the knot rubs against your love button while constricting his penis and scrotum (which can cause a harder erection). Yee-high!

4 Give your guy a demo of how you touch yourself when he's not around (it's a number 1 male secret desire). Start coy with panties on, flicking your fingers through the soft, silky fabric. Payoff one: He'll learn exactly how to press your buttons. Payoff two: You will be the reigning queen in all his future fantasies. **TIP:** To feel less like a solo act, include him – he can caress your other parts or he can give you his hand and you can use it how you like, making you queen for the day.

5 Attach a mirror to the ceiling above your bed for some voyeuristic fun.

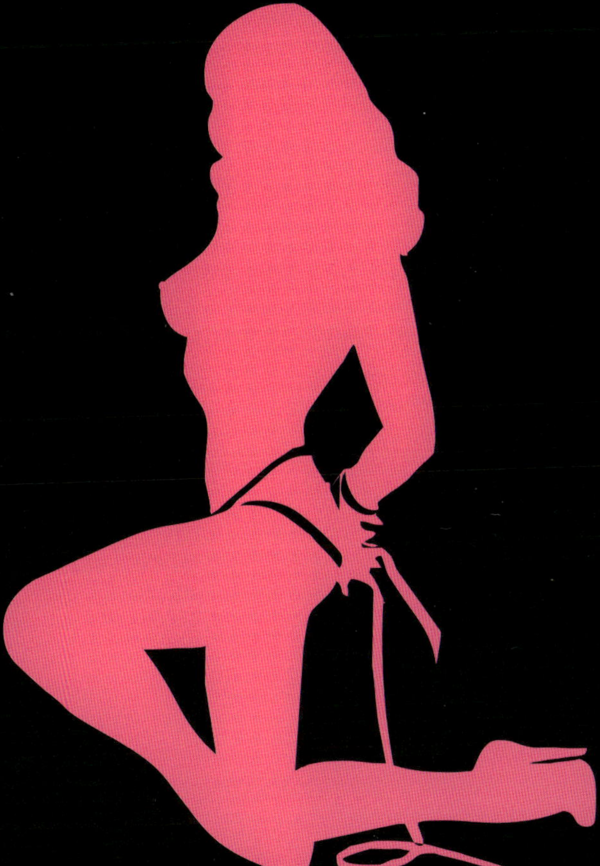

What to Wear, What to Wear

What makes on-the-edge clothes feel so extra-special sexy is that you can literally wear them anywhere. There is definitely a supermodel-thin line between what is high fashion and what is something you would find in a porn video – corsets, leather trousers, silky sheer shirts, lacy camisoles, fishnet stockings, PVC skirts and stilettos are just a few examples that have shown up on both sides of the style street.

All of which makes stocking up on your wardrobe a no-sweat, no-angst way to stretch your sexual boundaries. Read on for how to dress up your life.

Seven-Day Sinner

Put this on your daily agenda: Seven days of dressing up a sexy, sultry you.

MONDAY

AKA Moon Day. Wear white to work – but make it secretive, sexy, lacy white. Slip on a sheer white lace thong, a garter belt and a slinky white camisole under your usual work uniform; you'll feel like the drop-dead-gorgeous lunar goddess you really are! **S**

TUESDAY

This is your inner-tramp day. Do something naughty that you always fantasized about, but your shy side got in the way. Leave the panties at home. Instead, wear head-to-toe leather or PVC. If your workplace shuns the Harley-Davidson look, slip on a leather thong and bra or 'jumper bumpers' – small metal rings that fit around your nipple to keep them erect. **E**

WEDNESDAY

Mid-week – time to shake off stress, blahs and blues. In short, get a makeover. Hit a salon that can give your downlow region a new look. Hot pink dusted with glitter, royal blue with a white trim and lime green are just a few colours to dye for. If you can't get it done professionally, DIY with coloured mousse, gel or hair mascara that washes out with one shampoo. **X**

THURSDAY

The week is almost over, so what's a girl to do? Go shoe shopping. Find yourself the maddest, baddest sky-high stilettos you can. That extra six inches of height will transform you into a bona-fide dominatrix. To really get the kinks out, make them thigh-high and rubber. Now sashay your hot new self down the street. **X**

FRIDAY

The day of dressing sex-cess. Start the day in red – teddy, camisole, panties and/or bra. Then slip on a silk or velvet shirt that comes off with a quick flick of the wrist (velcro-tabbed or via snaps). After hours, pull out the stops – with cleavage down to here and a long strand of beads dangling in between. Later, just wear the baubles. As things heat up, use them to tease and please your lucky lad, running them across his skin and wrapping them around his limbs. Then roll them into a ball and knead his body into a state of bliss. **S**

SATURDAY

Get your booty shaking by giving him a lap dance. Do like the professionals do – Keep your guy fully clothed and make sure you're only wearing a G-string and heels. Absolutely forbid him to touch you (although you can touch him) – it'll give you a sexy, powerful feeling, and seeing your naked body but not being able to touch will make him crazed with desire. Straddle his legs, and wiggle your bottom. Grind slowly and seductively to the music, stroking your breasts, and making eye contact. Then mambo your way over to the mattress. **E**

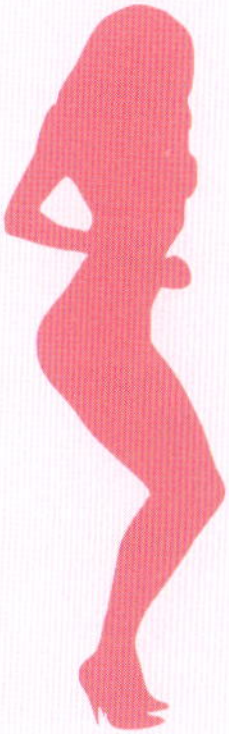

SUNDAY

Pour yourself into a sexy silky negligee and refuse to take it off (think of it as the reverse strip). He has to kiss and lick you through the fabric. **S**

Stripped Bare

It's not just what you wear – it's how you take it off. The last thing on his mind will be your cellulite. Promise!

★ Opt for an outfit that accentuates your assets. For example, if your breasts are best, wear a cleavage-catapulting bustier. For bottom babes, go for a bum-revealing G-string. **S**

★ So you don't pop out and knock him on the noggin, slowly slip down one bra strap and then the other before undoing your bra. **S**
TIP: Dangle the bra in front of him before dropping it on his lap.

★ Keep your heels on 'til the last minute. They'll lengthen your legs and make 'em look like something that's just strolled out of a porn flick. **E**

★ Wear stockings. You can give him a triple X view by sitting on a chair and lifting one leg at a time, then rolling the stocking s-l-o-w-l-y down with your palms. He'll be howling oo-la-la. **E**

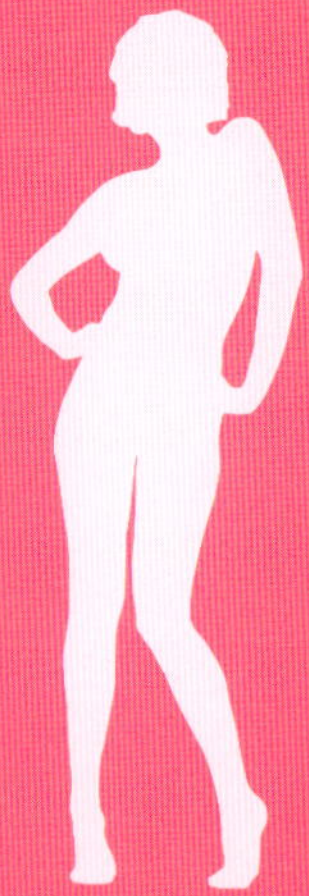

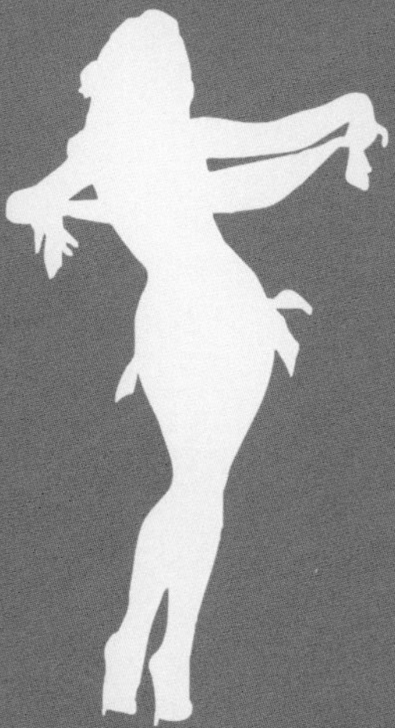

★ Drape yourself with feathery boas or silky scarves that you can slide off later in the show. **E**

★ Avoid these fashion don'ts when stripping.

- ♥ Tricky sleeve cuffs – undo them first so you don't have to stop when slipping your shirt off
- ♥ Tight-necked tops – you don't want to get stuck mid-strip looking more like a turtle than eye candy
- ♥ Elasticated waistbands leave very unsexy marks on the skin
- ♥ Back-fastening bras – front closers avoid any passion-killing fumbling
- ♥ Skip the suspenders (garters) – lace hold-ups are much less fiddly.

★ Try switch-hitting by stripping him. Slowly undo his shirt. Gently slide it off, kissing and licking his chest. Get down on your knees and remove his shoes and socks. Fondle his penis through his pants as you slip them off. He'll be putty in your hands. **E**

Hair Today, Gone Tomorrow

Tips for sexy head-to-crotch tresses.

★ Wig out. Try frolicking in the wig section of a department store. The payback for slipping on a totally new, man-made 'do? You can put on a different persona without much effort. Although you may, of course, need a fresh wardrobe to go with your sexy new alter ego. **E**

★ Dare to bare. Skip the usual bikini line trim and take it all off. Having nothing to cover you and buffer the sensation makes that area hypersensitive. And he'll love the fuzz-free access (more south-of-the-border mouth action for you). **X**

★ The best way to go hairless is to take a trip to your local waxing salon and let the professionals handle it. You can turn your expedition into a romp by taking him along. Some places even let him do the honours and pull the wax. Yeow – but at least he'll have an idea of what you're going through in the name of eroticism. **X**

★ If you opt to do it at home, turn it into a steamy love session. Light candles, prop yourself on the sink and spread your legs wide. He should take his own sweet time applying shaving cream. As he shaves you clean, he can slip in some teasing moves while whispering in a low, sexy voice how he's going to give you the best oral sex of your life. **X**
TIP: Old-fashioned switch-blades and disposable razors will give you nicks and burns. Use a safety razor, designed for female use.

★ Get creative and landscape your garden. Trim your hair into any pattern your heart desires: your boyfriend's initials, a lightning bolt, a butterfly – even an arrow pointing down (for the benefit of partners with no sense of direction). **X**

★ He can also go bald. A razor carefully taken to his little man and boys will make his penis look bigger by at least an inch or two. Not to mention that it'll prevent work stoppages when you have to pick the hair out of your teeth. **X**

Get the Hole Story

Buy your own personal love stud.

★ A tongue piercing can work wonders for oral sex by providing extra sensation to his frenulum and your clitoris (see www.safepiercing.org). Genital piercings also improve sensation. He can get his penis pricked, but rather than wait around for him to get over his wuss attack of letting people with sharp tools down in man-land, you can get a piercing like the 'triangle' which increases the sensitivity of your clitoris. **X**

★ A nipple piercing can turn your little bumps from something that felt OKish-nice to full-fledged erotic zones connected right to your nether regions. **X**

Clothes Encounters

Five fashion accessories no kinkster should be seen without.

1 Harness: This contraption lets you wear a dildo like a penis. Think of the endless possibilities – you can do him, he can double do you. **X**

2 Nipple clamps: If your nips have never felt that sensitive, this will be an eye-opener. You'll feel like there's an amazing livewire connection between your nipples and your clitoris. Start small with just the tip. You can always squeeze more as you play (although you shouldn't leave them in place for more than 20 minutes or you may cause injury). **X**

3 Vibroclips: These are nipple clips that add an extra kick of vibration. **X**

4 Nipple ring: Baubles for your bumps. He'll never snub your breasts again.

5 Orgasm balls: These small balls go clickety-clack inside your vagina all day (they are not worn during intercourse), keeping you on tingle alert. **X**

Playing with Props

Even the hottest couples can use some fresh, creative ways to keep their lust scorching. Luckily, there are plenty of fun accessories for raising the temperature available from sex accessory websites and stores. All you need is a little know-how and planning to get going. Get ready to lay on a red-hot, good lovin' party!

Get the Kinks Out

Sometimes you need to push the envelope to get the sex life you want.

GUARANTEED ORGASM BOOSTER: Strap on a hands-free vibe and feel your sex life soar. While you and he do the rocket jive, it'll give your – and his – lower regions a tantalizing tingle that will send you on a round-trip to the moon. **E**

GUARANTEED PENIS PROPPER: If he tends to droop, a cock ring will keep his package firmly in place. Get one with a built-in vibrator and you'll both be gyrating all night. **X**
TIP: Fit is everything. Go too loose and they do nothing; too tight and he'll never get soft (not as alluring as it sounds after two hours and a trip to emergency).

GUARANTEED MOOD SWINGER: Using edible body paint, scribble naughty words all over each other's bodies. Then lick it off. Use long strokes running the length of your lover's body. **S**

GUARANTEED PASSION ZINGER: Pick up an arousal balm and massage it on your most sensitive bits (nipples, inner thighs, genitals … you get the idea). They're spice-packed with mint or cinnamon and will give you a hot tingly sensation all over.
WARNING: A small amount goes a long way. **S**

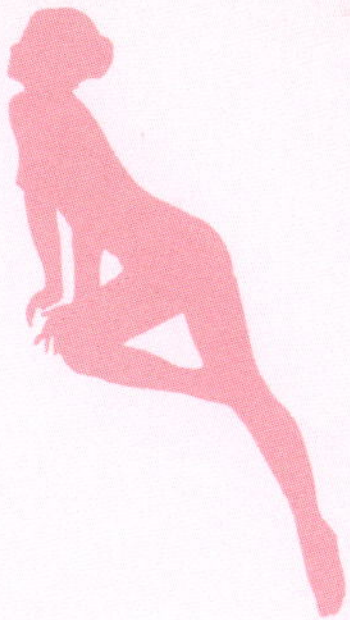

GUARANTEED POSITION PLEASER: Give any position a little oomph by stacking up some Liberator cushions (www.liberatorshapes.com). These cushions are designed to take the hassle out of new angles and moves. Plus you can take them anywhere, so no more out-of-bed rug burns. **E**

Hot and Handy Tools

How to play with your sex toys.

★ If your vibrator has two speeds, always start low so you don't jack the intensity too quickly.

★ When giving his popsicle a lick, rest your chin on top of a powerful vibrator to add an incredible buzz. **X**

★ Turn your scream machine into a sex toy for two. Slip it between your two bodies so it rests against the base of your pleasure switch during face2face loving. He'll be able to feel the vibrations while he's inside you. You'll both soon be pulsating with pleasure. **E**

★ Give him a tickle by stroking a happy trail with your vibrator from his lower belly to his inner thigh. Then lightly trace his love triangle, delicately stroking the head of his penis, moving down his shaft and gently circling his balls. Finish off by performing some mouth magic on him while grazing his twins and inner thighs with the vibrator. **E**

★ You'll be counting orgasms when he slips a dildo inside you while he's licking your lips. Especially if you look for one that's designed to rub your G-spot. **X**

★ Bring in a stunt double. When he needs a rest, he can fill you up with a dildo and then touch the base with a vibrator. Silicone is the most realistic material and also best for getting the vibrations to reach their target. **X**

Lubes, Oils and Salves

★ Instead of just going in dry on your next blow job, use a gel that not only gives him a high-pitched tickle but also gives your tongue a yummy razzah. Flavours range from minty to fruity so you can have a taste test. Unfortunately, it doesn't seem to have the same effect when the roles are reversed. **E**
TIP: Don't reapply the gel in an attempt to go the distance – it'll make your mouth feel like it's been to the dentist.

★ Make up your lips with some vaginal lip gloss and show him your best smile. He'll swoon over the different flavours and scents (and hopefully want to spend the whole night sampling them). **E**

★ Smear some fruit-scented balm on your nipples and you'll want to skip dessert and head straight to bed. These zesty creams warm to the touch and taste heavenly. **E**

★ Pour massage oil directly onto your lover's skin instead of on your hand first, as you would during a regular massage. He'll ooze from the sudden feeling of the cool massage oil and then the warming sensation of your hand rubbing the oil in. **E**
TIP: Massage oil is sticky so lighter is better (the last thing you want is a thick, slick coat you can scrape off with your nails). Also, use old sheets.

Anal Beads

★ Make it easy to go in or out by lathering up with plenty of lube. It's easier to pull out if you push down with your bottom muscles (as if going to the toilet). **X**

★ Don't get the bum's rush losing your beads. If your trinket doesn't have a ring or handle on the end, leave one or two beads outside the opening so you can pull them out. **X**

★ Timing is everything. Send your lover into a tailspin by s-l-o-w-l-y pulling the beads out during orgasm (they'll have to let you know when blast-off is, so you can start pulling). **X**

On the Menu

Put a little kink in your sex diet.

★ Have a feeding frenzy. Make an edible passion shopping list and then send your lover to pick up the booty. Suggestions: cake icing tubes to write on each other with, mints or pop rocks to tuck into your mouth for effervescent oral sex, ice cream to dab on and lick off hot bits, donuts to ring around his erect penis and nibble off, and Champagne for lapping out of your concave places. **S**
TIP: Chocolate does not wash off skin easily and leaves embarrassing brown streaks.

★ For chocolate lovers: When his penis is soft, run an ice cube over it and then cover it with chocolate syrup that hardens (available at any supermarket). Just make sure you suck instead of bite! **S**

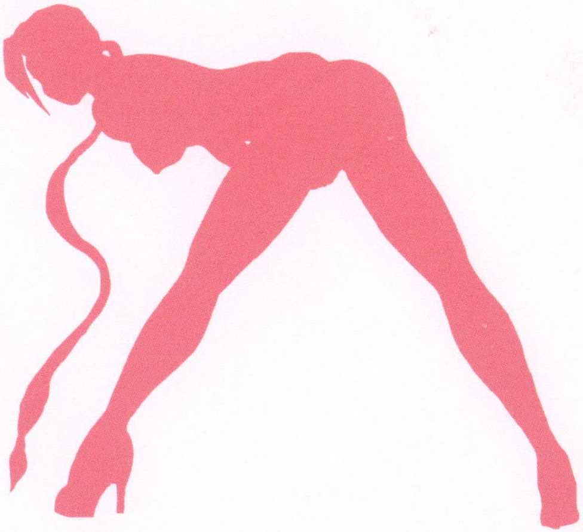

Household Goodies

Skip the toy store – here are nine things you have around the house to push your sex life to the edge.

1 A silk scarf can double up as a blindfold or an impromptu hand and leg truss so you can have your wicked way. **S**

2 A ruler or flat-headed hairbrush will transform you into the impatient teacher ready to discipline a disobedient student (or vice versa). **X**

3 An electric toothbrush can double as a his 'n' hers vibrator. Using soft bristles run it over your bodies, gently brushing the nipples and between the legs. Just be sure to change heads before brushing your pearly whites. **X**

4 Have a dust up with a feather duster – you can use it to apply honey dust or icing sugar to various body parts and then lick off your dirty work. **S**

5 Or pluck out just one feather to tickle your lover's bottom hole. **X**

6 Wrapping sheer, silky stockings around your hands like gloves will turn your hand 'job' into a pleasure. It's easier on you than using a dry hand and the sensuous fabric will make him crumple. **S**

7 Make an impromptu cockring by scrunching a fabric hairband around his penis base (not too tightly). It'll keep him in a state of suspended lust and the fabric will give a pleasure nudge to your love centre. **E**

8 Light an unscented, white candle (perfumes, colourings and beeswax all make the candle burn hotter) and tilt it above your lover's body to allow a single drop of hot wax to land on the skin at a time. For extreme thrills, alternate between hot wax and ice and slip on a blindfold so everything comes as a sexy shock. **X**
TIP: If you're planning below-the-belt drippings, shave first or die.

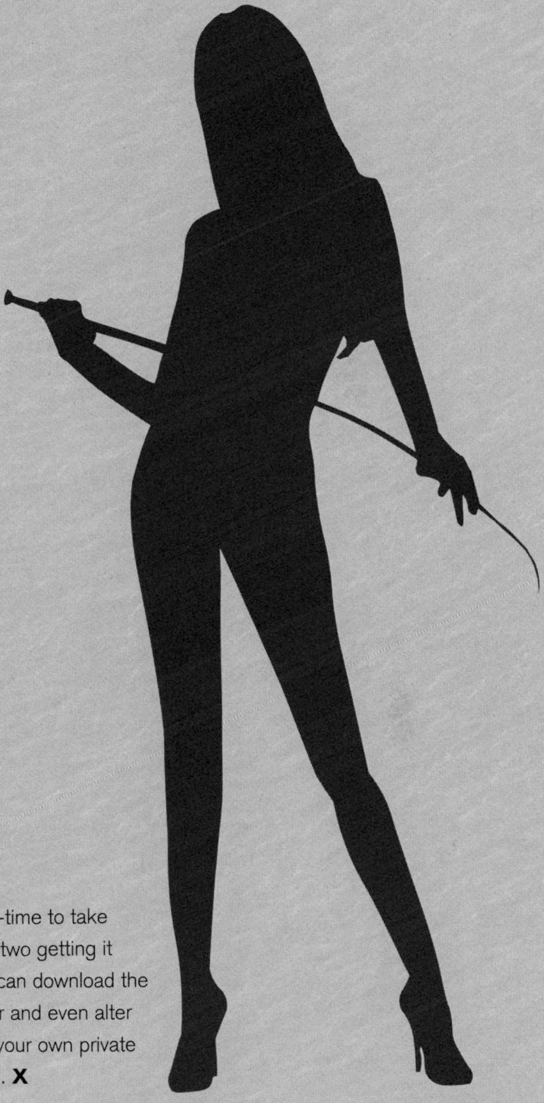

9 Set a camera on self-time to take sneaky snaps of you two getting it on. If it's digital, you can download the pics to your computer and even alter the images to make your own private x-rated blog paradise. **X**

Tease, Please

The fun starts here. You don't have to be into S&M to experience the pure erotic thrill that comes from playing tie-up games with your lover. Flexing your dominatrix muscles and calling the foreplay shots is a powerful turn-on. On the other hand, simply be a prisoner of your lover's lust and let them have their wicked way with you.

Don't worry. You won't need special equipment to get started (that's for later!). Just pack your imagination and the desire to romp rough. But remember: Sex, no matter how wild, is supposed to be about loving it up – not drawing blood!

How to Be the Boss in the Bedroom

Don't be skittish about telling your lover exactly what you want.

★ Play Lover, May I?. The rule of the game: No touching without asking, 'May I touch/lick/suck/bang your…' (insert favourite bit here). Naming the parts means you'll be forced to mouth off like porn stars. You can add a dom tone by establishing your chick-in-charge position and occasionally denying him access. **S**

★ Practise verbal bondage by telling him to act like a statue. He holds his hands up, each fingertip touching the opposite fingertip. Put a penny between each pair of fingertips so he's holding five pennies. Now order him not to let a single one drop, on pain of punishment (such as he has to be your sex slave for one day) and then go to work ravishing him.
TIP: This works best on a hard floor so you can hear the coin drop – which it definitely will. **E**

★ Don't give him a chance to think – straddle him, pull his head back with a tug of his hair and just take him. Use tough-love techniques like naughty ear and neck nips, pushing your fingertips deep into the fleshiest part of his buttocks while he thrusts, pulling his face to your breasts as you hit your passion peak. He'll be delighted with your diva moves. **E**

★ Swap roles and have him put on the bad-boy persona. Say you want him to take you on the rough side. His script: to pounce and hold you down, then breathe in your ear how hot he is (his talk should be part Romeo, part porno). Sex up the scenario by pretending to push him away, you damsel in desire! **E**

★ Lie back on the bed with your arms outstretched and purr, 'Do whatever you want with me.' **S**

★ Always cuddle after. **S**

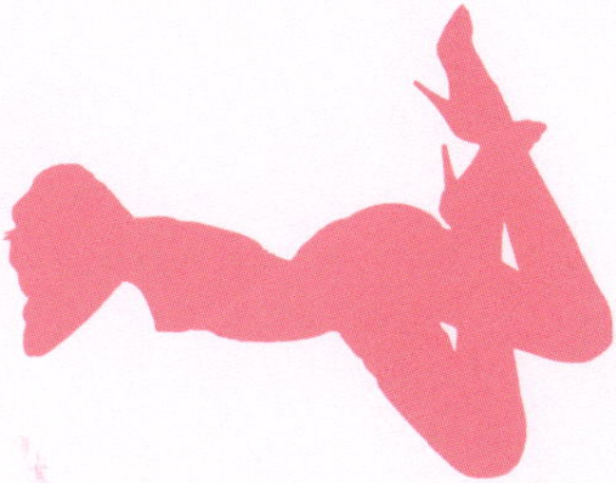

See No Evil

Give new meaning to the phrase, 'love is blind'.

★ Once you've got your man blind, treat him to a slew of new sensations: gently nibble him, trail your hardened tongue over his body, tickle him with your fingers, swish your hair over his bits. He'll have no idea where you'll strike next. At the crucial moment, climb on top, hold his face and make him stare right into your eyes as you ride him to oblivion. **E**

TIP: Start low-key and use your hands instead of a blindfold to cover his eyes.

★ Tantalize him by slipping a scarf over his orbs and teasing him any way you desire. You're in total control of his pleasure, so pull out the stops by stimulating him with sensual props. Mix up your touch to keep his temperature high. **E**

TIP: Don't forget to take a turn behind the veil so he can have fun ordering up your moans and groans.

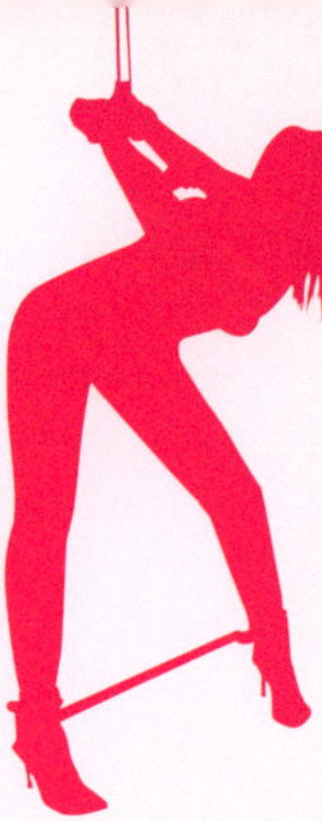

Get Fit-to-Be-Tied

How to tie one on and feel no pain.

★ When you're ready to be bound for love, don't reach for the handcuffs unless they're specially made for sex play (fur-lined, for example). The metal versions are more likely to bruise your wrists or – worse – break mid-play. The beginner's best is nylon because they open easily, and are affordable and comfy to wear. DIYers can use scarves, bandanas, stockings, a tie or cotton rope.
TIP: Always tie them loosely so you can get out easily in a pinch.

★ If your bed has no posts, you can wrap ropes around the legs of the bed and spread-eagle your lover. Or tie his wrists behind his back and then to his waist. **X**

★ Have him tie your hands and feet together and then set you up on your elbows and knees. He then comes from behind to worship you mercilessly while you love every minute of it. **X**

★ Tie him to a chair and then do a striptease followed by a lap dance (see Seven-Day Sinner on page 190 for how-to). **E**

★ Tickling is terrific torture that's especially good if he's all tied up with nowhere to go. Run a feather up and down his body until he begs for mercy. **S**
TIP: When he returns the favour, you may discover you're one of the few lucky women who can get tickled to orgasm.

★ One tormenting trick he can try on you: He ties you spread-eagled to the bed and rests a vibrator on your push button. While he plays with your breasts, you'll be writhing like a disco dancer trying to get the buzz exactly where you want it. **X**
TIP: To really put you into a Saturday night fever, he can switch-hit between an ice cube and a fur-covered mitt on your globes.

Spank Amateurs

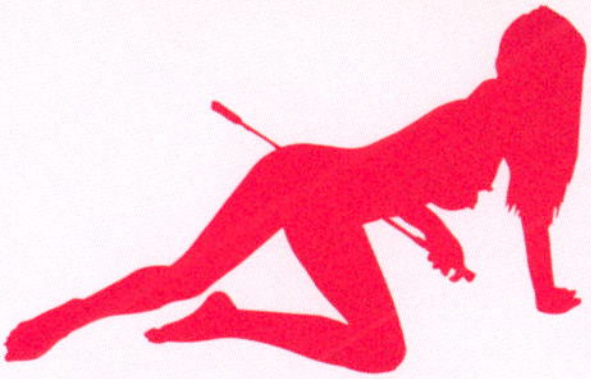

It's swattin' time.

★ Next time you're smack bang in the heat of things, whisper to your partner that you've been bad and you need a spanking. Add a little bottom squirming to emphasize your point. **E**

★ f you plan to be in charge of the smackdown, make sure he knows. Wear black thigh-high boots and a naughty teddy to set the mood and then tell him he's been misbehaving and needs to be punished. **X**

★ Get your lover in spanking position. The classic pose for her is bent over his knee with her bottom up for a good licking. If he's on the receiving end, he should lean against a waist-high object (table, bed, car) that'll brace him against her thumps.

★ Spank it like a pro. Your lover's bottom is not your boss's face, so keep your everyday aggressions out of the bedroom. Start by rubbing (you can rub one or both cheeks, but only smack one cheek at a time). Don't worry, before you know it, they'll turn the other cheek. After you smack it, rub the area a little bit, not only to soften the blow, but also to show that it was an affectionate butt whooping.

★ Hit the bull's-eye. The hind end's sweet spot is the well-padded bit where cheek meets the thigh. Spank close to the genitals and they'll indirectly get stimulated, sending your sugarbaby into sweet oblivion. **E**

★ Keep the rhythm. The winning beat is two light smacks, one slightly harder, then three light smacks and one hard one, and repeat. This build-up will deem you Spank Master. **E**

★ End with a bang. Spanking sessions end when the one on the receiving end cries, 'Uncle'. Ask, 'Will you be good now?' If they agree, lay off, kick back, and let them show you exactly how good. **E**

Pushing the Limits

Same time, same place, same position? Some fun and games can shake you out of your ho-hum routine.

Most of these tips take some preparation. But working a kinky act is never a quickie, which is why doing it makes you pant with lust. Deciding what secret desire you want to play out, stocking up on the equipment and planning the scene together are all part of the buzz. So shelve your inhibitions and get ready to vice things up with these sextreme suggestions.

Bottom's Up

The ins and outs of rear-ending in the bedroom. It's not a vagina; it doesn't secrete fluid. Unless you want to see your lover leap up and dig their nails into the ceiling, grease up. Silicone lubes (versus glycerine ones like K-Y and some versions of Wet and Astroglide) are slick and slidey and stay that way longer. For obvious reasons, it's a good idea for the partner on the receiving end to take a trip to the toilet (and possibly the shower for a soapy wash) before anything gets started.

★ You don't have to go for a deep plunge. The highest concentration of nerve endings is around the anal opening itself so just inch your finger or tongue in for a quick skinny dip while playing at the other end. **E**

★ The key is re-lax-ation. Start off with a long, warm bath, or better yet, give your lover a few teeth-numbing, stupefying orgasms before you head 'round back. **S**

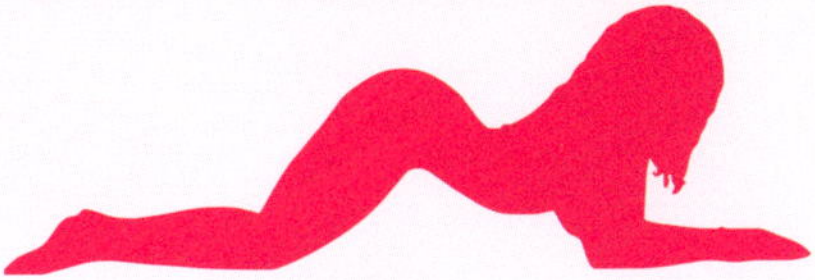

★ If you do decide to do a full bottom bungee jump, follow these four steps for a smooth dive.

1 Get cheeky. Don't lunge straight for the hole. Spreading and softly squeezing and rubbing your lover's derrière will put them in a relaxed, receptive mood. **S**

2 Test the waters with one, then two (well-lubed) fingers before you let little Johnny jump in. Work your way up very gradually, gently stroking the region right around the opening, then pushing gently at the centre but not actually penetrating. **E**

3 Get into position – puppy style is easiest for newbies. **E**
TIP: Hopping on top means you can call the shots but it tends to tighten your butt muscles, making penetration tougher.

4 Once the head of the penis is in, stop and relax for a couple minutes, to get used to the sensation.

★ Turn him into a love fool by poking his prostate (on the rectal wall on the side toward his genitals). Lick his lollipop at the same time and watch him drool. **X**

★ Try a little rim around the rosie with your tongue. Make your tongue flat and hard for the most yum-gasmic sensation. **X**

★ Toy with your bottom. Use a small dildo or vibrator specifically made for anal insertion (they're flared so won't get sucked in and lost in your no-man's land) or butt plug (a small flared stopper that's inserted and sometimes left in the bottom) or anal beads (think cheap plastic necklace – see page 196).

★ Use lots of hands-on techniques. While making a pass at the back door, work in a double play by slipping your other hand around the front end. He can use fingers or a vibrator on her orgasm lever or navigate his way down her vaginal canal, bumping along the bottom wall to buoy up the pleasure waves while she can pull on his boys or give his wood a jiggle. **X**

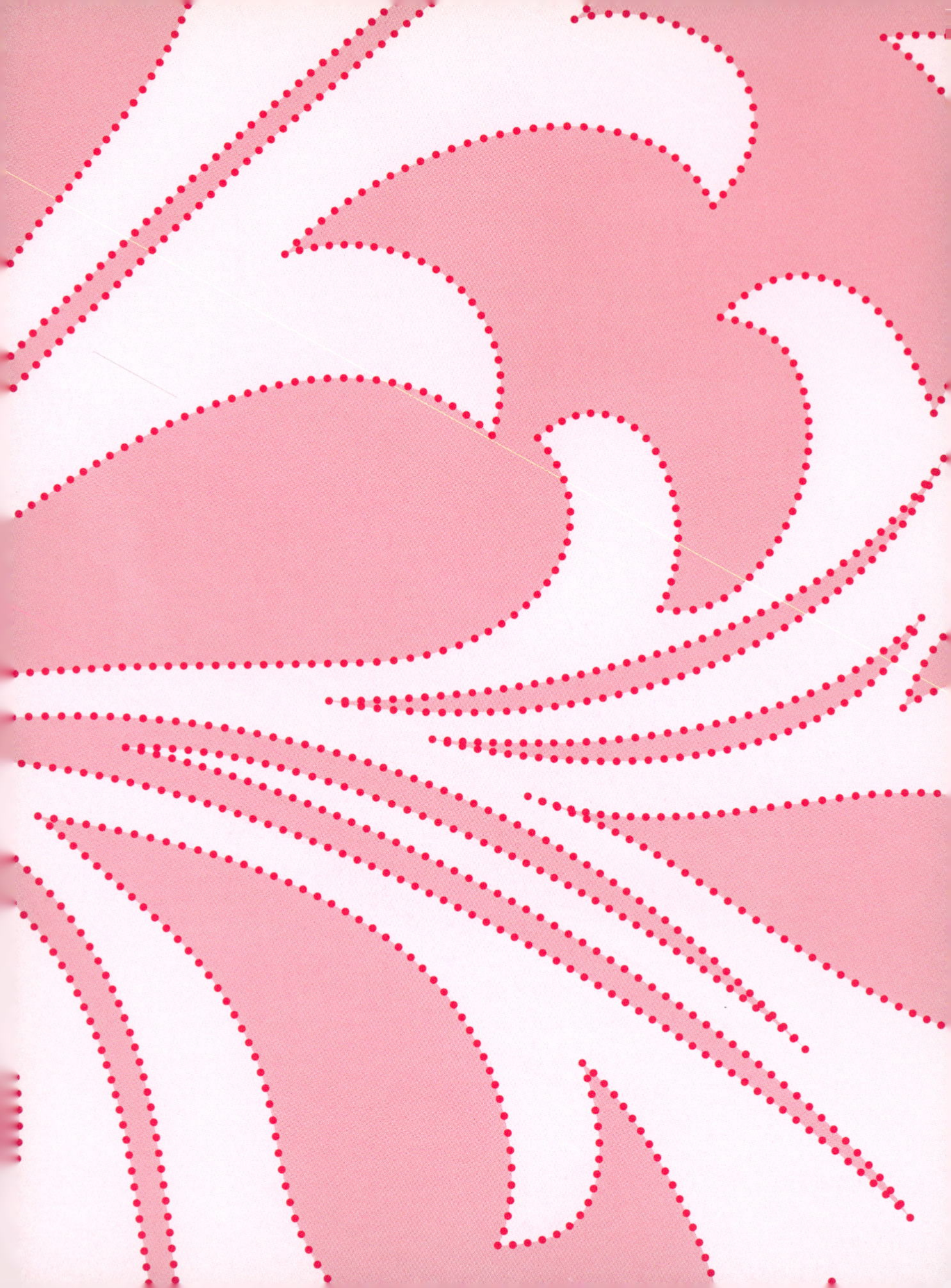

Chapter 8

Truly Astonishing Sex Tips

1 Eating chocolate can hike up your PEA count. Try smearing chocolate body-paint (available from sex shops) or chocolate syrup over each other's bodies, and then lick it off. Yum!

2 Scatter rosebuds over your bodies and the bed before you make love. The petals will become crushed between your sweaty bodies, gorgeously scenting your sex. Who said life wasn't a bed of roses?

3 Ask him to give you a belly orgasm. Sit erect on the edge of a chair. Your lover should stand behind you and place his hands, pointing downwards, in a triangle on your abdomen – and rub. You'll feel your ovaries get warm and tingle a bit. Breathe deeply. You'll soon begin to feel a sexy buzz.

4 Get some sleep. One study from an American sleep centre found that women who reported going to bed later than usual one night were rarely in the mood for making love the next. A possible reason for this is that when you're getting enough shut-eye, your levels of the stress hormone, cortisol, drop. Fatigue gives this hormone a chance to build up, which may erode sexual appetite.

5 Get him to tickle your Ahh! zone. Known as the anterior fornix zone, it's a soft, squashy bump located on the front wall of the vagina, between the G-spot and the cervix. This hot spot has awesome bliss potential – studies show that stroking here helps women to become easily lubricated and experience single or multiple orgasms during sex.

6 Wash each other's hair. Besides being incredibly sensual (think how good it feels at the hairdresser's), the Kinsey Institute New Report on Sex found that good grooming was even more important to lovers than penis or breast size!

7 Ears are an underrated erogenous zone. The lobe and the small area behind the shell have a hot line to the nerves. Stimulation from a darting tongue or a light, probing finger can be a powerful aphrodisiac – especially when combined with heavy breathing into the ear. Scientists call the phenomenon the auriculogenital reflex, and trace its origins to a nerve in the ear canal. Some men find it so exciting they actually climax from it.

8 Playing with temperature heightens the sensations because your blood vessels will alternately expand and contract. Run an ice-cube over each other's hot skin, or spray your sheets with ice-cold water.

9 Heat things up even more. Take a cup of hot fruity tea to bed with you, sip it and then wrap your mouth around your lover's most sensitive parts. Ask him to do the same. You'll melt with pleasure.

10 Say 'Ooommmm'. In one study, meditation breathing and relaxation exercises significantly raised levels of dehydroepiandrosterone (DHEA), the hormone that revs up our sex drive.

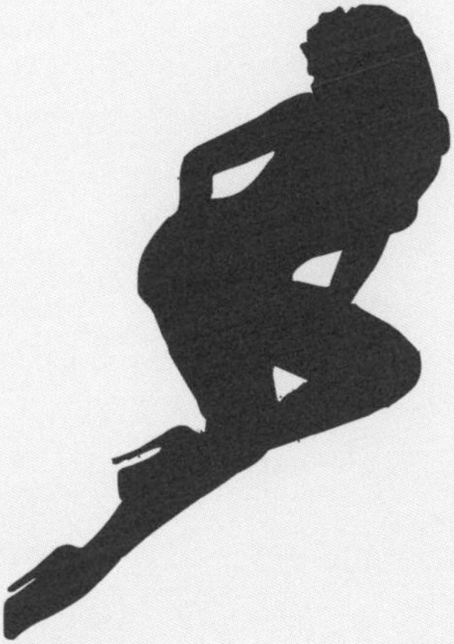

11 Masturbate. It's a delicious cycle. The more frequent a woman's sexual activity – alone or with a partner – the better her sex life. Research has found that women who pleasure themselves regularly have increased sexual desire, more orgasms, greater sexual and relationship satisfaction and higher self-esteem. Makes you want to give yourself a hand!

12 Prime your body for a hot and heavy love session. Power squats will build up the muscles that are exercised during sex, giving you added stamina for the main event (your orgasm). Stand up, feet slightly further than shoulder-width apart, arms straight out in front of you for balance. Push your hips and bum back, and bend your knees forward (no further than your toes). Then straighten your legs. Do three sets of 15 reps, three times a week.

13 Tickle the roof of his mouth with your tongue.

14 Give his sacrum a stroke (and get him to return the favour). This small dent, located just above the crease of the bum, (aka the Bermuda Triangle of love) is extremely responsive when massaged in a circular motion with your thumb.

15 Come – er – prepared. Red-hot lovemaking is a sure thing if you keep your libido on a low boil throughout the day by fantasizing about body-bonding with your lover later on. One study by the Center for Sexual Health at Tulane Medical Center in New Orleans, found that when women have a mental rehearsal for sex, especially if they have a history of orgasm no-shows, their bodies become more sexually responsive within 30 seconds, once the action really gets going.

16 Resist the urge to make love for a few days, and then set an exact date and time to break the fast. In the meantime, tease each other mercilessly with deep kissing, erotic massage, and light stroking, especially on your favourite hot spots. Sometimes, building anticipation is the most glorious foreplay of all.

17 Learn how to tell a farmer's-daughter joke. Research by the Society for the Scientific Study of Sex found that women who see the funny side of life, and are amused by sex-related jokes, are lustier and have higher levels of sexual satisfaction than their more serious sisters.

18 Call in late to work. The prime time for him to have sex is 9 am. This is when his testosterone level peaks, so physiologically it's all systems go. (You'll probably feel more in the mood, too, as a woman's testosterone cycles often echo her partner's.)

19 With more than 72,000 nerve endings, your hands are very receptive sex tools. Make the most of every single nerve ending by putting on blindfolds and caressing each other from head to toe, lightly tickling with your fingertips, kneading with your fingers, pressing with your palms, circling with your whole hand and patting gently with the sides of your hands.

20 Make things sizzle by coating his testicles in minty toothpaste before intercourse. The ever-increasing heat sensation this produces will make you both squirm with pleasure. Afterwards, you can lick off any residue (although it won't help to prevent cavities!).

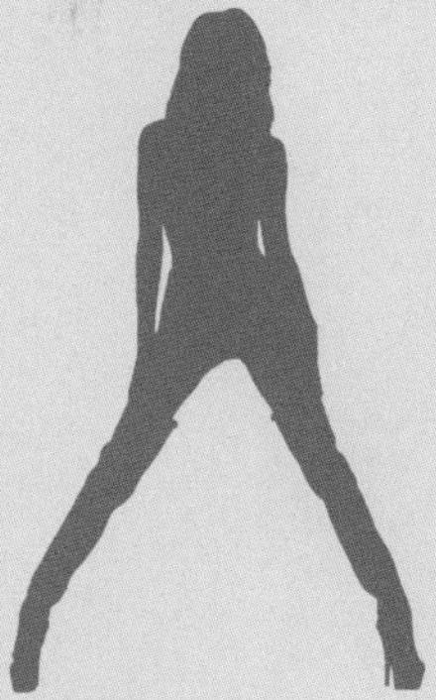

21 Give him a kiss he'll feel all the way down to his toes. Lie facing each other and press your lips together tenderly à la Clark Gable and Vivien Leigh in *Gone with the Wind*. While you can keep the connection for as long as you want, Tantric teachers recommend you hold it for at least seven seconds, in order to experience an all-over glow.

22 Ignite a secret hot spot. Because urine is expelled through the urethra, we don't usually think of this tiny area of tissue just below the clitoris as a sexual point, but Kevin McKenna, PhD, an associate professor of physiology and urology at Northwestern University Medical School, found that it's a possible trigger for orgasm when pressed. It's also a good place to shift your lover's attention, post-orgasm, when your clitoris feels too sensitive for direct stimulation, but you're still in the mood for pleasure.

23 Give each other a body-to-body rubdown: ask your man to lie face down on a soft supportive surface like the bed or a thickly carpeted floor. Start crawling on top of his back, rubbing it with the front of your body and hands. Work your way downwards, finishing with your breasts wedged in the crease below his buttocks and your genitals somewhere mid-leg. Your clitoris will sizzle from the pressure of your movements, and the sensation of your breasts on his bottom will tantalize him. If you do this immediately after bathing while your bodies are still moist, it will make things sensually slippery, without losing any of the fabulous friction.

24 Even the shade of your boudoir or lingerie can affect your rapture rating. In a study at Loyola University in New Orleans, both sexes thought that the three most erotic colours (in descending order) were red-orange, dark blue and violet. And the least erotic? Grey.

25 Style your pubic hair. But instead of a complete shave with a razor (which can leave a decidedly un-sexy itch), trim each other with electric clippers. **BONUS**: the vibration from the clippers will add a delightful tingle. If he's not sure he wants a haircut down there, tell him that the shorter the hair, the bigger his organ will look.

26 Touch for your own pleasure, not your partner's.

27 Act like a vampire and go for the neck. (Do NOT draw blood!) Gently kissing and sucking the points to the immediate left and right of the Adam's apple drives 1,000 volts of pleasure through the spine.

28 Have a two-in-one orgasm. Some sex experts believe we experience two types of orgasmic sensations – the first is a sharp twinge that occurs when the clitoris or base of the penis is stimulated; the second is a warm melting feeling that happens when the inside of the vagina or the shaft of the penis is aroused to climatic heights. Experience both types, one after the other in a single love fest, and you've had what's called a blended orgasm. He caresses your clitoris until it's almost too sensitive to touch; then he moves his attention to the interior of your vagina. Once you are feeling totally aroused, he moves back to your clitoris. Meanwhile, you are doing the same with his penis, moving from the base to the shaft to the head, and back again. Keep on going for an hour of mind-warping climatic bliss.

29 Rub a few drops of lavender oil into your hair. According to the Smell and Taste Treatment and Research Foundation in Chicago, this scent turns men into lust-crazed beasts (or near enough). Your olfactory turn-on? Cucumbers (no phallic jokes, please).

30 Take your vitamins and minerals. According to nutritionists, vitamins B and E and zinc enhance the efficiency of the nervous system, leading to a stronger libido and better orgasms.

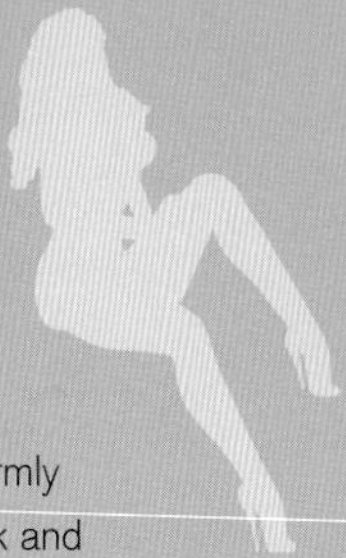

31 Rub his inner G-spot. Get him to lie on his back. Sit between his legs and massage the shaft of his penis with one hand, using lots of moisture and a circular stroke. When he's getting close to orgasm, use your other hand to caress his perineum firmly (the hair-free patch of skin at the base of his scrotum). Sit back and watch his toes curl.

32 Ask your lover to give you a three-finger caress. By bringing together the pointer, middle and ring finger of his hand, he will be able to massage every sensitive nerve ending on your clitoris.

33 For a more intense orgasm, lie on your back with your head lower than the rest of your body, either by lifting your hips with your hands, with the help of some supporting pillows under your hips, or by positioning yourself so that your head hangs slightly off the bed. This increases blood flow to your brain and changes your breathing, both of which can add to arousal.

34 Try *dok el arz*, which means 'pounding in the spot'. An ancient Arabian position, it manages to give him the deep penetration that he desires, and your clitoris the attention it craves: the man sits down with his legs stretched out, the woman then places herself astride his thighs, crossing her legs behind her man's back. Lining things up, the woman guides her lover into her. She then places her arms around his neck while he embraces her waist and helps her rise and plunge upon him.

35 Light a candle. Undress. Explore each other for as long as the candle burns. When it sputters, go for your climax in the dark.

36 Comedy isn't the only thing that requires good timing. Pencil in sex during the four days following ovulation (around the third week of your cycle), when your testosterone levels peak. Studies show that women are more likely to masturbate, initiate intercourse and reach orgasm easily during these days (caveat: they are also more likely to get pregnant).

37 Give each other an alternative orgasm by stimulating one of these acupressure hot spots: use the heel of the hand to gradually increase pressure in the centre of the crease where the thigh joins the front of the torso, rub the area between the mid-thigh and the genitals, or use a forefinger and index finger to massage the temples in gentle circular motions.

38 Spice up foreplay with the alphabet game. Take turns making capital letters with your tongue very slowly on each other's genitals. You might make it to 'M'…

39 Pump it up. Your heart, that is. Thirty minutes of aerobic exercise three times a week can do wonders for your sex life – and your orgasm power: studies show it boosts testosterone levels (making you more in the mood for sex), tones cardiovascular endurance (enabling you to last longer), increases blood-vessel diameter and blood volume (making vaginal tissue more sensitive), and improves circulation (making orgasms more forceful).

40 Remember to breathe. According to a study by the Center for Marital and Sexual Studies in Los Angeles, most women tend to unconsciously hold their breath during sex, which kills arousal. Instead, try taking slow, regular breaths as you feel your excitement build. The more you can control your breaths, the deeper your orgasm will be.

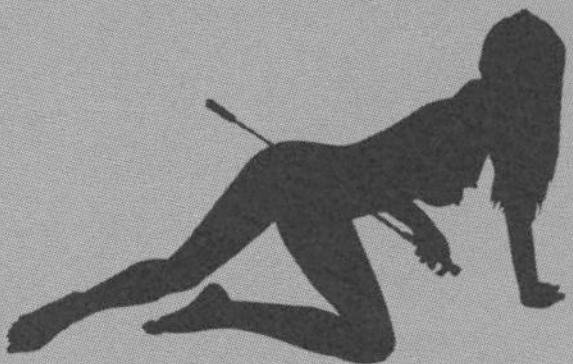

41 Having a sexy dream at night can make you sizzle during the day. With practice, you can induce a siesta orgasm by indulging in your favourite turn-on before you start counting sheep at night.

42 Feed each other an ambrosial fruit salad. According to the Smell and Taste Treatment and Research Foundation in Chicago, oranges increase penile blood flow by 20 per cent, strawberries spur sexual satisfaction, and spices like nutmeg and cinnamon make you want to do it again and again …

43 Play some Harry Connick Jr. A study from the National Opinion Research Center in Chicago found that jazz listeners had the most sex. The fluidity of the music also makes you move more rhythmically – especially when you're horizontal.

44 The biggest problem with orgasms is that his erupt speedily while yours come at a more leisurely pace. But you can keep him to your rhythm with a tender tug. Using your thumb and fingers, encircle his scrotum (not testicles!) as he nears climax. Squeeze firmly and pull down lightly for a few seconds. He'll groan with ecstatic pleasure if you do it right, with pain if you are too rough. So remember to take it easy – practise makes perfect.

45 Introduce him to your breasts. According to a survey in the *Practical Encyclopedia of Sex and Health*, only 50 per cent of women say they enjoy having their breasts fondled during foreplay – mainly because they're in the hands of men who fumble the ball. Tell him what pleases you by putting your hand over his and caressing the area together.

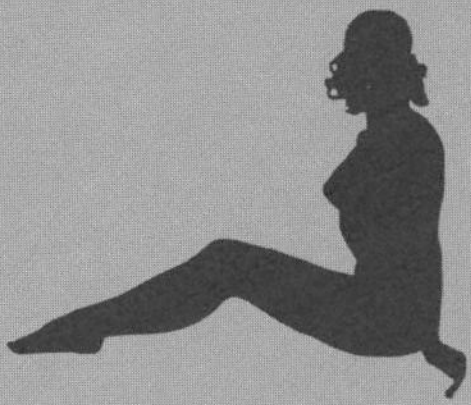

46 Exchange tongue baths – starting from the fingertips, lick each other's bodies all over, leaving not a single patch unwashed.

47 Do one thing differently. If you normally nibble his ear, nibble his nipple. If you always end up on top, do it lying on your sides. An *Archives of Sexual Behaviour* study showed that making one small variation in your standard sex routine can help lovemaking to become thrilling all over again.

48 If you're almost at orgasm and get stuck, sex researchers Julia Heiman and Joseph LoPiccolo have found that deliberately tensing your legs, stomach, arms or feet will send you over the edge.

49 Check *Old Moore's Almanac* for the lunar schedule. A report published in the *New England Journal of Medicine* states that women are 30 per cent more sexually active (read: more likely to rip his clothes off) during a full moon than at any other time of the month.

50 According to Masters & Johnson, orgasms are really just a sweet release of incredible tension. So boost the intensity of yours by hovering around the 'Ohhh-I'm-almost-there' spot for as long as possible. Get as close to peaking as you can, then relieve the pressure by getting your lover to stimulate a less sensitive area of your body. Repeat until you're ready to burst.

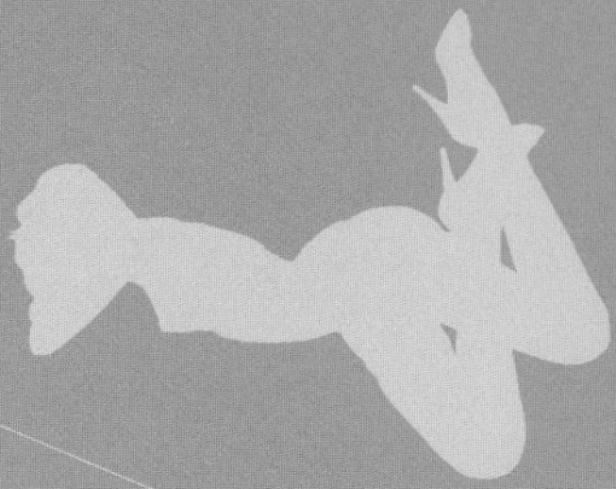

51 Have him lick your upper lip. Just about every ancient Eastern sex philosophy claims that this site is the key to a woman's clitoris, and touching it is guaranteed to create cosmic sparks.

52 Forget oysters. The best aphrodisiac (although, perhaps not the tastiest) is a diet low in lard. The lower your body fat, the higher your levels of testosterone and DHEA. Low blood-cholesterol levels can also reduce plaque build-up in the arteries, increasing circulation and blood flow to the genitals. Bon appétit.

53 Read any Harold Robbins' book. Rent a sexy video like *Bitter Moon* or *The Lover*. Racy images jump-start your sexual response by raising levels of phenulethulamine (PEA), carnal chemicals that flood your brain when it's buzzed on sex.

54 The penis has its own hot spot just waiting for the right touch. The raphe is a seam, which you can both see and feel, that runs lengthways along the scrotum. Hit his moan zone by lightly tracing your fingers along the line, moving from his bottom forwards and up towards the base of his penis.

55 Go straight to sleep. Sex in the middle of the night, after you've both clocked up a couple of hours' shut-eye, can be much more profound.

56 Time your foreplay. A Kinsey report found that only 7.7 per cent of women whose lovers spent 21 minutes or longer on pre-penetration fun and games failed to reach orgasm.

57 For an indirect pleasure prep, gently press the area about 6.5 cm (2½ inches) below your belly button for about three minutes. This helps promote blood flow, which stimulates the entire pelvic area. Oh, and you can expect a mind-blowing orgasm, too.

58 Ribbed condoms are supposed to add to a woman's pleasure. But turn one inside out and those little ridges can do wonderful things to his penis, too (mix in a dab of water-based lubrication to avoid breakage).

59 Skip the perfume wrist spritz. In Ayurvedic medicine, the ancient Indian science of health and healing, the lower stomach is considered to be the centre of a woman's sexual stamina. Dabbing the area with fragrances that are supposed to have aphrodisiac qualities – such as neroli, jasmine, sandalwood and patchouli – will set the scene for a steamy night. As you become aroused, the increased blood flow to your pelvis generates heat in the area, helping to release the fragrance – and unleash your animal magnetism.

60 Get hot – literally. Soak in a warm bath, take a steam or Jacuzzi at your gym, sunbathe (slap on the SPF first), jump up and down until you're sweating, make love on sheets fresh from the dryer. According to a Czechoslovakian study, heat depletes our body's store of stress hormones, making us more in the mood for *l'amour*.

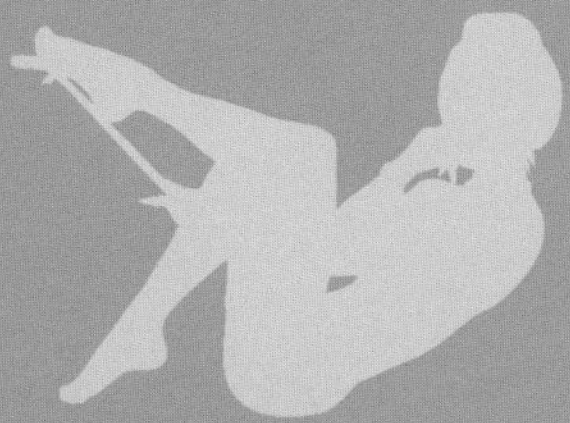

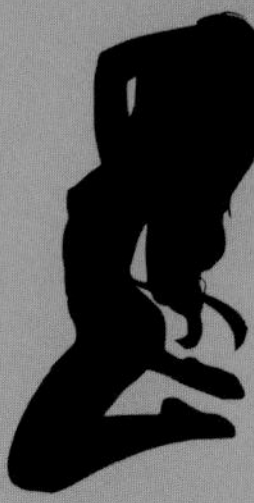

61 Climb on top when making love. Experts agree that when a woman is in this position, three marvellous things happen: the forward-facing wall of the vagina (the epicentre of all of her genital hot spots) and the clitoris are more easily stimulated; she can control the angle and depth of penetration more easily; and she becomes more involved in the act of intercourse – all of which add up to a more achievable and impressive orgasm.

62 Buy a porn flick. Yes, YOU. An *Archives of Sexual Behaviour* study found that women get just as turned on watching erotica as men do. However, since most of the films available are for the male market, you might want to check out Femme Productions, which produce films specifically for women and couples.

63 Blow his … mind. Put both of his balls in your mouth at once. Use one hand to circle the top of the sac, and gently pull it down to bring the balls together into a neat swallowable package. Being extremely careful to cover your teeth with your lips, take the sac in your mouth and give him a tongue lashing he'll never forget.

64 Anthropologists call a reddened mouth a 'genital echo', a term that includes all body parts with a passing resemblance to a love organ. Drive the point home by applying some bright red lipstick and giving him a blow job (making sure he has a good view).

65 Equip yourselves with torches and turn off the lights. Take turns turning the high beam on each other. Whatever part of the body is lit up has to be caressed for five minutes with the lightee's mouth or hand.

66 Sex in the bath can actually dry out your juices. If you're not using latex birth control, add a few drops of oil to the water to keep things lubricated.

67 More thrusting does not necessarily mean more fun. The most sensitive nerve endings in the vagina are actually near the opening, so shallow penetration is really better for you. Since this also allows constant stimulation to the head of the penis and, specifically, the hypersensitive frenulum, both of which are squeezed by the vaginal muscles located near the vaginal opening, you won't hear any complaining from him, either.

68 During foreplay, pull back your hair so that he can see your face.

69 Try something new three times. The first time, you may be worrying about bending your knees, elbows or both at the proper angle; the second time, you will be thinking about how to make it work for you, but the third time you try you'll probably find that you're able to relax and go with the flow.

70 Give each other a deep tonsil-touching kiss, every time you meet. Experts agree that smooching can be more intimate than sex (which may be why prostitutes often draw the line at kissing). When psychotherapist Sylvia Babbin, PhD, investigated the number of times an average couple kissed, she counted only four-and-a-half pecks per day – including hello, goodbye, good morning and good night.

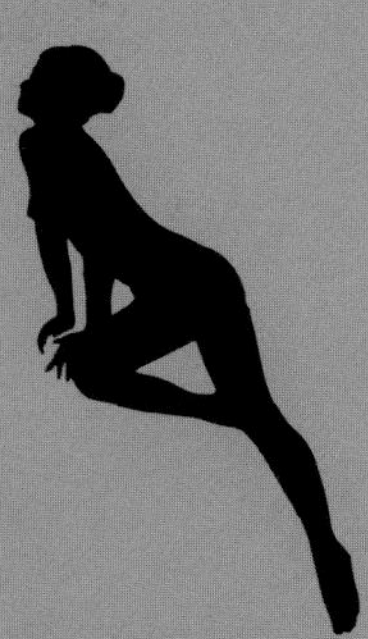

71 Deep-throating is a learned technique. To swallow his penis as fully as possible during oral sex, throw your head back as far as it will go. This opens up the throat and allows you to accept an elongated object without causing your gag reflex to react. Lying on your back with your head over the edge of the bed and breathing through your nose is the most comfortable way to maintain the position.

72 Make him stand to attention. A study at a recent American urology conference established that taking 80 mg of ginkgo biloba a day can boost his potency (and your pleasure). Seems the herb increases blood flow by relaxing the arteries. But don't expect overnight results – it can take several weeks before you notice a difference.

73 Move in together. A national survey of Family and Households found that men and women who live together have the most sex, making love more often than non-cohabiting couples, even after they marry.

74 Make intercourse clitoral-friendly. Research shows that only about 30 per cent of women have regular orgasms from penetration. But when they use something called the coital alignment technique, the odds improve to 77 per cent. Begin with your man on top in the missionary position. He should then slide slightly forward, causing his pelvis to override yours. Instead of thrusting (and completely bypassing the clitoris), you rock your pelvis up while he responds with a downward pressure, so the penis shaft stimulates the clitoris directly, and possibly the G-spot, too.

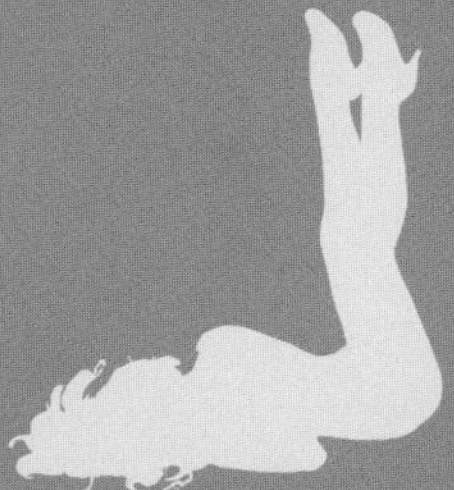

75 According to the Kinsey Institute, the average man thinks about sex at least once every half-hour. Use this knowledge!

76 Ride a roller coaster – or anything else that makes you quake with fear. According to research conducted by psychologist Judy Kuriansky, PhD, for Universal Studios Amusement Park in Florida, experiences that make our stomachs flip over result in a surge of adrenaline and endorphins, which can make us feel more lusty.

77 Reorganize your bedroom for a more amorous atmosphere. According to feng shui, the ancient Chinese art of creating a harmonious living environment, if your bed has a view of the whole room, with nothing blocking the door, your lovemaking will buzz with energy and understanding.

78 Telling a man you want him is the sexiest thing you can do. It packs the same erotic punch as informing him that his team's won, he's won the Lottery AND you've bought him a Harley Davidson. You don't have to be obvious. Simply turn a hello peck into a mini make-out session, and he'll soon get the picture.

79 Go to the pub. According to research cited in *Nature* magazine, one to two glasses of alcohol elevates testosterone levels in women – especially women who are ovulating or on the Pill. But get him to stick to water – booze has the opposite effect on male testosterone levels.

80 Emptying your bladder makes it easier to stimulate your G-spot.

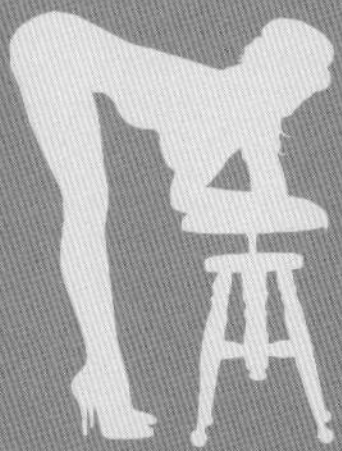

81 Here's a good argument for investing in a nicotine patch: a new study reveals that quitters have more orgasms than when they smoked. Tobacco chemicals supposedly constrict blood flow to the vagina and penis, and may lower testosterone levels.

82 Unlike women, men don't have built-in lubricants. Give your hand a lick before caressing his penis to help make things deliciously squishy.

83 Get him to pay as much attention to the minors as the majors. According to a study by the Kinsey Institute, 98 per cent of women say they are as sensitive to having the labia minora, the delicate inner lips that surround the clitoris, stroked, as they are to direct clitoral stimulation.

84 Teach him how to multiply. A study from the Health Science Center at Brooklyn found that men can actually learn to climax and keep their erection through three to ten orgasms. The key lies in helping him raise his orgasmic threshold by constantly stimulating him until he's a heartbeat away from ejaculating, then stopping and resting before stimulating him again. The results should be explosive.

85 Get your tongue pierced. Apparently the stud is perfectly positioned to give extra friction on the most sensitive genital bits for men and women. Of course, you could try and create the same effect by slightly air-drying your tongue and sticking a frozen pea to it.

86 Masturbate in front of each other and find out what really turns you on.

87 Make the missionary position work for you. Start by changing the angle of his dangle so that his penis pushes up against the front wall of your vagina and tickles your G-spot. This can be done by slipping a small pillow under your hips or having your lover place his hands underneath your hips and lifting your whole pelvic area.

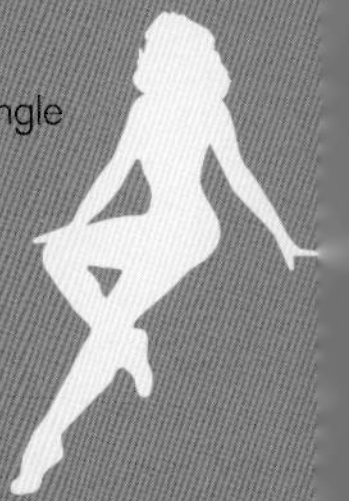

88 Show yourself. Men like to see naked women, which is why newspapers with topless models continue to flourish (although he STILL says he buys them for their thought-provoking articles). According to the US National Health and Social Life Survey, 50 per cent of men aged 18–44 find watching their partners undress 'very appealing'. Only vaginal intercourse ranked higher.

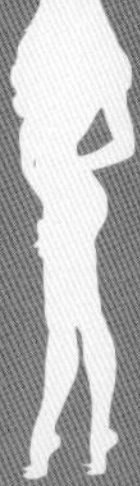

89 Plan a romantic rendezvous in October. This month sees the annual peak of testosterone in men, which explains why July (nine months later) is the busiest season for obstetricians.

90 Condoms don't have to interrupt your fun if you make putting them on a part of foreplay. Hold one very gently in your mouth, with the opening facing out. Then, using your tongue to help, gently roll it down your lover's penis with your lips (covering your lips with your teeth will prevent tears to the latex).

91 Access your sexual chi (energy) by practising the following ancient Indian breathing technique: block off your left nostril for 15 minutes (if you don't want to use your finger, a piece of cotton wool will do). This should redirect your airflow and ventilate the left side of your brain, which supposedly controls sexual arousal and creativity.

92 Have him try the 'Venus' the next time he gives you some oral stimulation. Ask him to alternate between lightly nibbling your clitoris, and flicking his tongue rapidly back and forth over the area. The result is a peel-you-off-the-ceiling kind of orgasm.

93 Make him climax faster than you can say, 'Fellatio'. While sucking his penis, squeeze your thumb and index finger in an up-and-down motion along the ridge on the underside of the penile shaft. Then, using the same two fingers, squeeze under the sac of his balls, with each finger manipulating a ball in the same up-and-down motion (imagine you're milking a cow). You'll produce an orgasm with the intensity of two in a row.

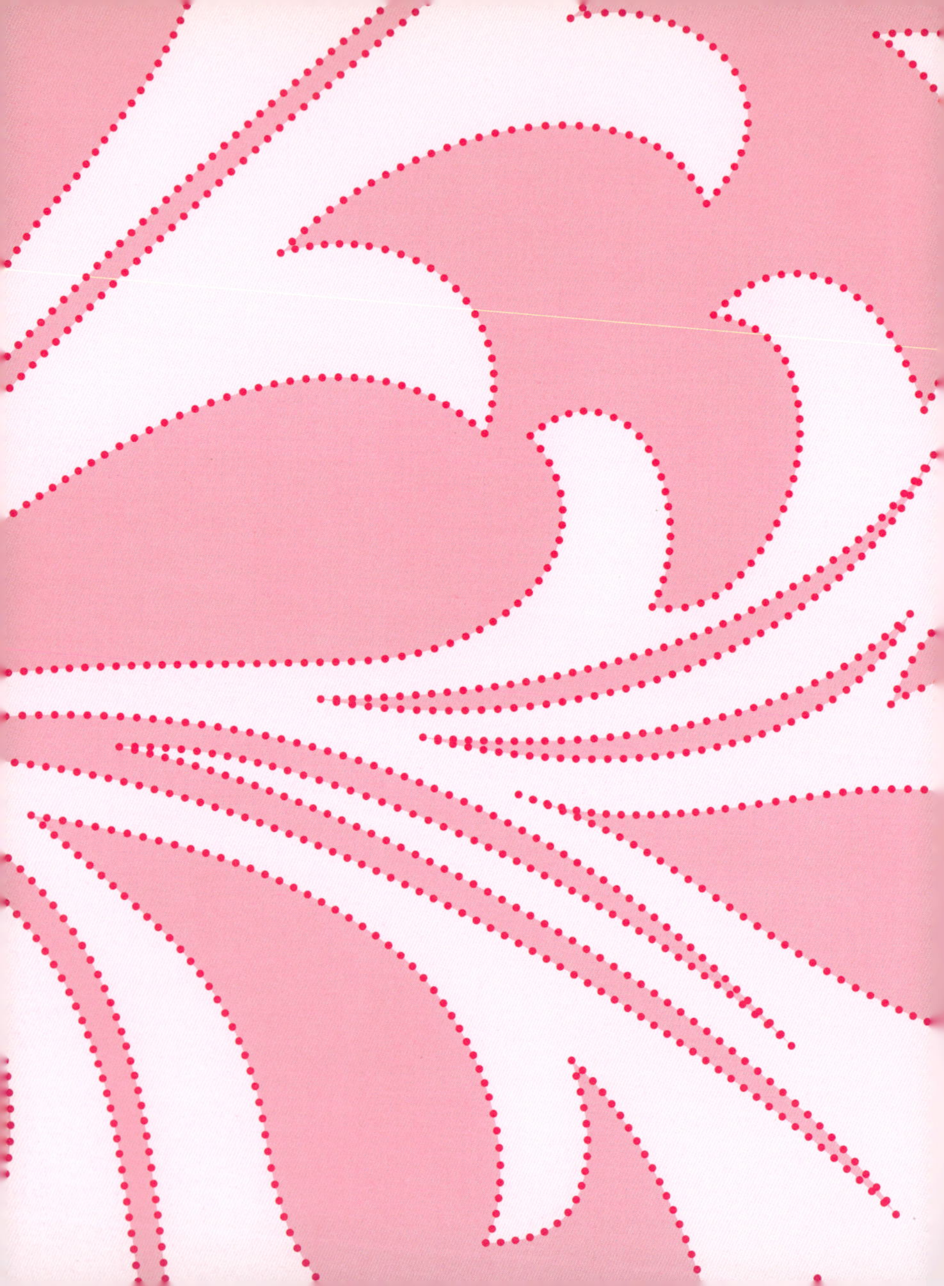

Chapter 9

Break-Ups

Denial

This isn't happening to me.

Studies have found that it doesn't matter if you are the dumper or dumpee – EVERYONE has to go through emotional phases similar to grieving in order to deal with relationship meltdown.

The first stage is denial. As in, 'Huh? I didn't see it coming. OK, things haven't been working out for a while, but it's not like he's an axe murderer.'

The reality is, unless things are blatantly bad – he's hitting you, cheating on you with everything on the planet, wearing your clothes – it can be hard to be 100 per cent positive that this guy isn't your Mr Right. Even then, you may think, 'Maybe this is just a rough spot that we need to work through,' or, 'It's me – I'll change and things will get better.' Odds are, once you're feeling this way, they won't. Here's how to tell where to draw the line.

Over and Out

Seven swift ways to figure out if he's the real deal or if the two of you are history.

1 You're starting to abhor what you used to adore. A University of Ohio study found that there's a flip side to love in that the things that first attract us are often the very things that start turning us off when the relationship is skidding towards a dead end. So his sexy take-charge attitude now seems controlling. Your fun-loving 'life of the party' suddenly seems more like an odious flirt. And his charming romantic streak begins to feel needy and insecure.

2 You argue over who started the last big fight.

3 You're putting up with behaviour from him that you wouldn't normally tolerate from a bank teller or shoe salesman, let alone someone you supposedly love. Research by relationship guru Barbara De Angelis, PhD, has found that women – especially younger ones – are easily susceptible to the myth that Love Conquers All and will, therefore, stay in a relationship way past its prime in the hope that the man will (miraculously) change (see tips 15–19 for other bogus true romance beliefs).

4 Love him/Dump him

- ♥ You have good sex together regularly/The only thing that's good about being together is the regular sex.
- ♥ He's yours/He's there.
- ♥ Looking at him, you think, 'How did I get so lucky?'/Looking at him, you wonder, 'WHAT was I thinking?'
- ♥ You know no-one will ever love you like he does/You fear no-one will ever ask you out again.
- ♥ His screensaver is a picture of you/His screensaver is a picture of a naked woman (not you).

5 A man from your past shows up and, even though he's straight out of jail, you don't hesitate to straddle his Harley.

6 You don't panic that he may be flirting with his new assistant at work (the one you know for a fact is an ex-porn star).

7 You hate the way he breathes.

Don't Get Burned

Seven secret signs your man is about to bolt.

1 He's been criticizing you big time. According to communication experts, this is the typical male way of saying, 'I'm not really interested in you anymore,' while justifying his decision to bail. His secret wish? That you'll get so fed up, you'll say, 'I'm outta here.'

2 He introduces you as his 'friend'.

3 He asks you if you have ever thought about having an affair (translation: he's thinking about it).

4 He suddenly starts making nice with you. According to a Texas Christian University study, there's a break-up blueprint that most people follow when they're getting ready to dissolve their partnership: you notice other people, you guiltily try to make things lovey-dovey with your own partner, you get pissed off with the effort, repeat the cycle twice and then call it quits.

5 You notice a dramatic shift in your sex life. If you did it a lot, you now do it less, and vice versa. An *Archives of Sexual Behaviour* study discovered that the former happens because he's getting it elsewhere (or fantasizing about it); and the latter because he is desperately trying to make things work out.

6 He suggests a repeat performance of that time you had amazing sex in the lift (elevator) – only you've never had sex in a lift.

7 He won't make plans for the future, even for tomorrow night. Research on men and communication confirms what you knew all along: guys are notorious for not breaking bad – or ANY – news. To avoid confrontation, he might stop talking, calling or e-mailing, or move to another city – anything to keep from telling you he wants out. If you do corner him, he's likely to stutter and stammer, make a joke out of it or blurt it out in a way that feels like a groin kick from Jackie Chan.

Once Upon A Time

Unless you want to become the heartbreak queen, erase these love myths from your heart.

MYTH: You think he is the only one.
REALITY: Wrong. There are millions of potential soulmates for every person in the world.

MYTH: Your heart will never fully recover.
REALITY: It will.

MYTH: True love conquers all.
REALITY: True love doesn't conquer a lying, cheating bastard or even a Mr Not-Quite-Right who is perfectly sweet but leaves you yawning.

MYTH: 'If only I were prettier, thinner or smarter (or whatever!), it would have worked out.'
REALITY: You might be Gwyneth Paltrow's more gorgeous cousin who could kick ass on the Weakest Link and he'll still dump you if he wants out of the relationship.

MYTH: When you have incredible body-melting sex with someone, it must be love.
REALITY: When you have incredible body-melting sex with someone, it must be a great orgasm.

Bargaining

Should you let him go? All you want to know is what you can do to stop the pain. NOW. You have reached stage two.

Obviously, it's always better to be the leaver than the leavee. First of all, because it's going to be more of an ego boost to be the one who is doing the dumping rather than the one who is getting dumped. But also, you need to be the one to call it a day if you think you might have even a remote interest in getting your ex back sometime in the future.

A slew of studies on the perverse workings of the human mind have found that we are more likely to want what we cannot have. Ergo, leave him and you instantly become catnip for him. So here's how to let your man know that he is about to rejoin the singles world.

The Blow-Off

A clean break is all in the timing.

AFTER A FEW DATES

THE METHOD: Become the invisible woman.
HOW TO DO IT: If you've just had one date, don't answer his calls or e-mails. He'll either (a) forget about you, (b) meet someone new or (c) assume you've been kidnapped by a cult. If you've had a few more dates but aren't really a 'relationship' yet, allow so much time to pass between dates that in the interim travel agents have started selling trips to Mars. Do this by screening your calls and hanging out where he doesn't.
KEY PHRASES: If he happens to catch you unexpectedly, simply say you're so busy right now that you don't have time for anything but work. For the truly dense, you may have to use the 'I've met someone else' line.

AFTER A FEW MONTHS

THE METHOD: Give him the old 'It's not you, it's me' speech. Polls show that although this is the least-used method, it's the most effective, as it keeps things from getting personal and therefore reduces the risk that he'll start hurling 'big ass' insults.
HOW TO DO IT: Rehearse what you are going to say in advance. This will make it easier to keep to your script and not get sidetracked into unseemly 'discussions' about the size of his genitals (you) or your eerie similarity to your mother (him). Sit him down in a public place, such as a park (he's less likely to cry, beg or get violent). Avoid restaurants and pubs (he may retaliate to your dump method by dumping food or drink over your head).
KEY PHRASES: 'I'm not ready for commitment' or 'I want to concentrate on my career' are both hard for him to argue against. Another possibility: cite irreconcilable – and, if possible, irreversible – differences, such as his religion, profession, race, height and/or country of origin.

AFTER ONE OR MORE YEARS

THE METHOD: Draw it out (but not for so long that the break-up lasts longer than the relationship itself). This way, you work through your guilt, fears of being alone and the habit of the relationship before you actually spend a night as a newly single person.
HOW TO DO IT: Have Discussions About The Relationship. Drop not-so-subtle hints about how you are losing interest. Talk about the things that really bug you. Pick fights, then say, 'See? We're incompatible.' (WARNING: This last one doesn't work with boyfriends in the mental health field – they'll simply call you passive-aggressive and hoodwink you into going to couples therapy.)
KEY PHRASES: 'I think we should see other people.' Also good, 'We can still sleep together' (there's no reason why you shouldn't get some good sex out of a bad break-up, but use this line only if the sex is really – REALLY – incinerating).

Make Him Suffer

According to research by Charles T Hill, PhD, of Whittier College, California, the quickest way to wound a guy where it hurts (read: his babe-magnet abilities) is to dump him.

LET HIM GO GENTLY: Butter him up with more flattery than he gets from his mother. Telling him he's a great person who will make someone very happy someday will make him feel so good he'll be eager to forget you and get on with wowing the rest of the female population.

PRICK HIM: Tell him you just want to be friends. Then offer to set him up with one of your friends, mentioning she hasn't been in a relationship for a while. He'll hear: (a) you see him as a sexless hang-out buddy, (b) who is not capable of getting his own dates and (c) is only fit for desperate women.

MAKE HIM CRY: Sleep with his best friend or brother. Remember that the best way to achieve a 'clean break' is to make it as harsh as possible, so the parties involved don't ever get to see each other again, partly due to sheer embarrassment and partly due to the restraining order.

Speak Out

DECIPHER HIS FAVOURITE EXIT LINES

'You're much too good for me.' READ: 'You're not the one.'

'I'm under a lot of pressure right now.' READ: 'I don't find you sexy any more.'

'I like you too much.' READ: 'I'm scared to get involved.'

'You're too together to put up with my crap.' READ: 'You're boring, I'm history.'

'I'm not ready to get serious.' READ: 'I am but not with you.'

IF HE BREAKS UP WITH YOU,
SOCK IT TO HIM WITH THESE SURVIVOR LINES

'Phew. Now I don't have to confess about the affair I've been having.'

'Cool. I just met a hot guy and was wondering how to break it to you.'

'So now would not be a good time to tell you I've decided to become a lesbian?'

'Guess I won't be giving you that secret Eastern oral sex technique I learned as a surprise for your birthday.'

'Tell the truth – you're doing this because you feel bad that you've never been able to give me an orgasm, right?'

THESE SNEAKY BREAK-OFF TACTICS ARE SO DEVIOUS,
HE'LL THINK THE BREAK-UP WAS HIS IDEA

- One night in bed, after a particularly hot-and-heavy session, murmur in his ear, 'I've always wanted five kids – what about you?'
- Pick, pick, pick on your soon-to-be ex-lover until he can't wait to leave.
- Become impossibly demanding, selfish and possessive until he loses all interest.
- Smother your partner with love – call him ten times a day, insist on spending every waking moment with him, and tell him he is your life. He'll be gone before you can say, 'You complete me.'
- Tell him that you have decided to become a born-again virgin and plan to hold off on sex until you get married.
- Get caught with your pants down.

Breaking Up Is Hard To Do

If you're too chicken to say the words yourself, try one of these ready-made aids.

★ Send a card that 'bulls-eyes' your I-love-you-not message. Simply handwrite a personalized message and on-line greeting card company www.sparks.com will send it for you via regular old snail mail or e-mail. For those who prefer the cut-and-dried method, try this message: 'Although our lives have only crossed each other's paths for a short period of time, I can already tell you this … it's been long enough.'

★ When you want to avoid that I-wish-I-said-that feeling, log onto the Cyrano website at www.nando.net/toys/cyrano.html. They'll write a personalized goodbye for you based on information you type in. Easy-peasy.

★ If the indirect approach is more your style, send an anonymous note and a trial-size bug repellent through the post, direct to his door.

★ If Romeo needs things spelled out more clearly, visit www.dfilm.com, where you can single-handedly produce a digital, animated short staging your break-up scenario, complete with soundtrack.

★ Tell your boyfriend you have to talk. Then put on Paul Simon's 'Fifty Ways to Leave Your Lover', Carol King's 'It's Too Late' or Nancy Sinatra's 'These Boots Were Made For Walking' and walk out the door.

★ Say, 'You'll be needing this' and give him one of Melissa Etheridge's early CDs.

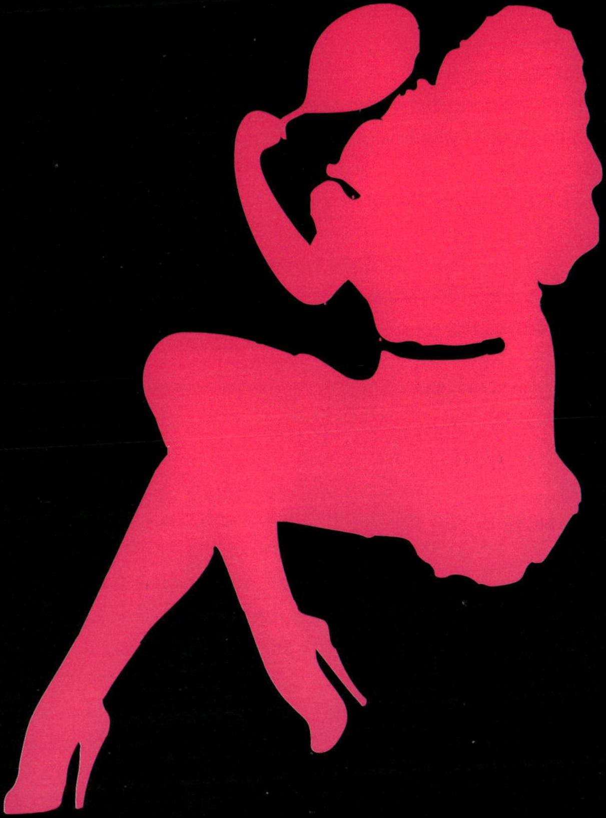

Depression

I can't believe this is happening to me.

You've just entered Splitsville (population: you). And it hurts bad, even if you were the one who downsized him. That's because breaking up is more than just saying goodbye. It's easy to delete his number from your speed dial; it's a lot harder to get him out of your heart. Researchers at the Medical College of Virginia have found that no matter who dumped who, your likelihood of depression rises 1,130 per cent after the end up of a relationship. Hello, stage three!

Bottom line: recovery isn't going to happen overnight. Truly getting over someone takes effort. Here's your plan for getting him off your mind – and having a little fun at the same time.

Total Rebound

Follow this guide to help you dry your tears and survive the first 24 hours.

★ All you want to do is sit alone on the floor with a candle burning and Toni Braxton wailing 'Un-break My Heart' on the stereo. So go ahead – brood over him, linger over every detail of the relationship. Many people ignore or deny their pain, pretending they're doing fine. Big mistake. Psychologists have found that you need to give in to your misery now, so the feelings don't drag on and on and invade every future relationship you have with other guys, with your friends, or even with yourself.

★ Weep. Snivel. Blubber. According to an Oklahoma University Health Science Center study, crying lowers blood pressure and relaxes muscles, making it a great natural tranquillizer for reducing physical and emotional agitation. But only if you tell someone about your sorrow as soon as your tears have dried.

★ Take heart. The more you hurt, the better a person you are. One study found that it's the truly 'good' people – trusting, vulnerable and loving souls – who are the ones that really hurt when a relationship ends. Another upside – these are also the people who get a lot more out of life than the people who claim they've never had their heart broken.

★ Take out your calendar and choose a date to end the pity party and pull yourself together. Research has confirmed that you need to set a deadline to your emotional torment before getting on with repairing your heart (turn over to the Fix Your Heart – Fast section, pages 240–2, for some quick remedies).

★ Take the sad song cure. Play Sade, The Smiths, Alanis Morissette – any music that gives the illusion that the whole world understands how you feel right now.

★ As for 'your song', avoid sobbing whenever you hear it by giving the song a new memory. Play the song with some good friends and dance on tables, stand on your heads – do anything that will make you burst out laughing the next time you hear it.

★ Throw an Ex Party. Rule out anyone handing out 'you'd feel better if you got out of bed' advice (you won't). You want sympathetic souls who will listen to you endlessly recount every detail of the break-up. Let them dole out tissues and cookies, tell you you're right, that you're not getting stress zits, remind you that you're a totally smart, fab babe and give you shoulder rubs (all that tension from crying!).

★ Don't call him. No ifs, ands or buts. Even if you broke up with him. If he calls you, don't pick up. Studies have found you need at least a one-week breather before sane talk is even possible.

★ Use cucumber slices or cold teabags to reduce the puffiness around your eyes. Drink lots of water – it will make you feel less dehydrated after crying.

★ Do not – DO NOT – phone him. Especially after drinking five Cosmopolitans. Set all your speed dials to your best friend so if you do try and call him, you'll end up ringing her (she can then remind you that it's over and you are way too good for him).

Fix Your Heart – Fast

Follow these tips to learn how to bounce back and jump-start your life (and heart) again.

★ Focus on today. Take things one step at a time, one day at a time. Relationship experts say that if you start looking towards or thinking about next week, next month or next year, you'll feel overwhelmed.

★ Set aside a period of time each day for grieving. You're allowed to wallow in self-pity between, say, 7 and 7.30 every evening. If you find yourself thinking about HIM at 9.13 am, tell yourself you'll think about that during the allotted time.

★ Don't lie in bed all day fantasizing about the last great orgasm you had with him.

★ Adopt a pet. Experts say that interacting with pets can reduce blood pressure, increase the rate of healing and ease depression. Pet therapists use animals to help alleviate these symptoms among critically ill patients, and there's no reason why you can't get the same benefits (if it was a nasty break-up, adopt a pit bull terrier and take him for frequent walks around your ex's block).

★ Give yourself a pinch for every negative 'No-one will ever love me again' thought. This process is called retraining your brain. Ouch.

★ Give yourself one week to indulge – eat nothing, eat just Ben and Jerry's, go out and party, go on a shopping spree (with HIS credit cards), flirt with the postman, have (protected) meaningless sex. Then stop and reassess. Studies show this cooling-off period will help give you distance and perspective.

★ Scribble down all your heavy thoughts in a journal. It's like having a 24-hour therapist – someone to listen without interrupting. Alternatively, turn your pain into fiction. Just imagine: 'He' ends up losing his job, his hair and the woman he left you for, while 'you' meet a tall, handsome stranger who has a PhD, a six-figure salary and an even bigger heart. (Check out *Heartburn* by Nora Ephron if you want to see how you can make money from anguish.)

★ Put your pain in perspective. Listen to country music or watch a daytime talk show (in your current state of mind, you'll be able to totally relate).

★ Go on a chocolate diet. Chocolate contains a natural amphetamine, phenylethylamine, the same one our brains produce when we fall in love and that makes us feel giddy and elated. When we fall out of love, we have PEA withdrawal.

★ Just Do It. You probably don't much feel like breaking a sweat, but research shows that working out for just 30 minutes a day is a major mood-buster (and gut-buster if you've been on a chocolate diet). Your body starts pumping out endorphins, those all-natural feel-good chemicals which not only kill your pain, but also make you feel inspired, strong and chock-full of self-confidence (plus you'll look fabulous if you run into him again). BONUS: pretend the ball you're hitting, the punchbag you're slugging or the pavement you're pounding is his face.

★ Put a positive spin on what is happening. You may feel rejected and a failure because your relationship has disintegrated, but for every drawback there is an advantage. Don't think of it as a 'failure', but a 'transition'. You aren't 'abandoned' or 'left behind', you are 'ready for something new'. Write down all the negative statements that occur to you, and then rewrite every single one of them with a positive slant.

★ Call up an old friend who used to have a crush on you for a confidence-booster.

★ Weekends are tough for the newly single woman. Form a Saturday Night Club and have a standing date with a bunch of similarly solo friends.

★ Reprogramme your thoughts. Stop mid-sentence if you've been obsessing about what you could have/should have/would have done differently. Instead, change your chant to what you can't/won't/ shouldn't ever do or take in a relationship again. The point? When you check out what happened or what went wrong in a relationship, you can figure out how to try to make sure it doesn't go wrong again, or if it does, to at least (hopefully) recognize it when it's happening (or, you can just blame him).

★ Give yourself six weeks. According to studies, this is about how long it takes to get over a severe loss.

★ Vow NOT to swear off men. Research has found women who avoid any emotional attachment after a bad break-up are much more likely to leave or destroy their next relationship for fear of getting hurt again.

★ Wait at least 90 days before having sex again (think of it as your ex-relationship's warranty). Apparently, researchers have found that this is enough time to let your body get charged up for sex again.

★ Send his stuff packing. Studies show that we get physically addicted to the pheromones secreted by the person we sleep with. So by cleaning the house, you're psychologically telling yourself that you are making room for something (or someone!) new.

★ Walk past a construction site once a day.

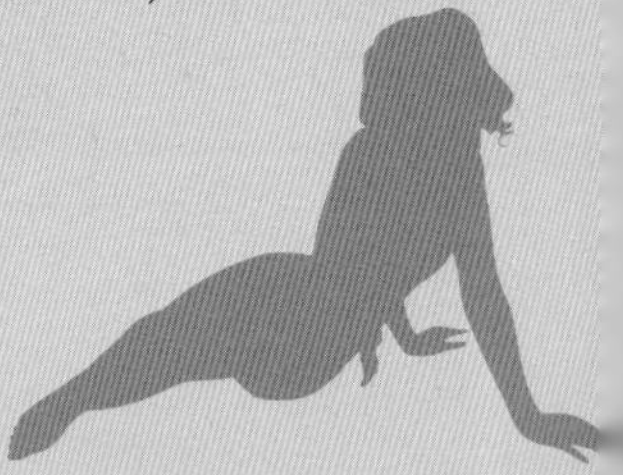

Social Ruts

Match your mood to your support system.

★ Visit your mother if you want to be babied and cooked your favourite foods.

★ Find your dad if you just want to hang out silently with someone and maybe hammer a few things.

★ Call your best friend when you need to hear how sexy, smart and wonderful you are.

★ Get together with a happily married couple if you need instant proof that being back with the 'singletons' is better.

★ Gather single girlfriends when you're ready to go prowling for fresh meat and have catty bitch sessions about your ex (they've been there, done it and bought the T-shirt).

★ Dial male friends when you need reminding that not all men are swine.

★ Look up an old ex for a passionate fling.

★ Get in touch with his friends when you need to let out all the venomous things you have ever felt about him. It should (a) get back to your ex and (b) allow you to gauge whether the listener likes or dislikes your ex, perhaps giving you something in common in case you wish to make him suffer (see page 234).

Ex Head Out

Exorcise your ex for good.

★ Replace the photograph of him next to your bed with one of your precious pooch.

★ Make a list – yes one of THOSE – about everything that was bad about the relationship (be honest!). He nagged you. You didn't trust him. You didn't have a lot in common. You get the picture. Carry the list for the next few days to get you over the 'I want him back' hump. Refer to it as necessary.

★ Insert 'bastard' (or some similar epitaph) every time you say or think his name.

Anger

Why does this have to happen to me?

This is the 'Arrgh! I'm so mad I could spit' stage. Bitterness and regret rule as you obsess how you gave this man three good dates/months/years – time that could have been spent doing … well, other things. With other men! You're not sure with whom, but they would have been awesome. Instead, you were working like a dog to build something real and lasting with that (fill in appropriate noun). Well, if he thinks he can treat you like that, forget about it.

The thing about anger is that you need it for recovery – experts have found that a little outrage goes a long way towards stimulating adrenaline, making you feel stronger and more confident. The danger is that you can get so stuck in your 'he loses his hair/job/life' fantasies that you don't move on with your own life.

Don't fight your rage; feel the pain, but direct it. Here's how to get mad, get even and then get over him.

Revenge is Sweet

Make him pay without risk.

★ You may think you need to trash him to move on. But according to research, getting revenge is exactly what prevents you from moving on. Apparently, every second you waste focused on him is one second less that you are going to feel better. If you can't help yourself, learn how to get revenge without leaving a trace.

★ Write a hate letter to your ex. Then destroy it. Repeat as often as necessary.

★ Get together with your friends and, using a doll, hold a mock funeral for him. Or destroy his photo, slowly ripping it as if you were tearing out his heart.

★ If you must get him, keep it legal. Call and tell him you have an STD (this is a double whammy because he'll think you were cheating on him). Get him a personal ad, saying he prefers 'full-bodied,' older women. Report all his credit cards as stolen. Sign him up for every piece of free junk e-mail under the sun. If he doesn't change his phone security code (and who ever does?), check his messages and delete any important ones (translation: those from women and bosses).

★ Check out these ultimate revenge websites; they'll do all your evil work for you:
www.virtual-design.com/demos/voodoodoll: Design your own virtual voodoo doll to torture and e-mail him the gruesome playback.
www.flwyd.dhs.org/curse: When you've run out of every four-letter word in your vocabulary, pick one from the Elizabethan Curse Generator.
www.anonymizer.com: Send all the vicious stuff you want and NEVER get traced.
www.dogdoo.com: Get down and dirty and send him virtual doggie poo.
www.deathclock.com: Find out when your ex's time on earth is up.

★ Plan your revenge in detail. Psychologists say that, for example, dreaming you called his boss about him skimming money on his accounts so he gets fired without a reference, never gets another job, ends up homeless and alone, etc., is better than actually doing it. It reminds you that you have the power, girl. You just choose to use it only for good.

★ Use your pain and get creative. Alanis Morissette hit it big with her Grammy-winning song 'You Oughta Know' about getting dumped; Carly Simon grossed $2.5 million from her song about a vain ex-lover; Ivana Trump has made millions playing the trump card after The Donald left her for a younger model; and Mia Farrow received $3 million for trashing her life with Woody Allen, after he left her for her adopted daughter.

★ Know your local revenge laws; it could serve you well. In Singapore, a 32-year-old woman who made more than 60 crank calls a day to her ex's fiancée was fined almost £5,000 for harassment.

Ex-Files

Your manual for surviving sickeningly common close ex-encounters (no tissues required).

THE SITUATION: ARRANGING TO RETURN EACH OTHER'S PERSONAL STUFF AFTER THE SPLIT.

DO: Make a list of everything that's yours and tell him he can do the same. If you don't think you can maintain your cool, get a friend to do the drop-off for you. Alternatively, arrange a blind drop-off in front of each other's homes.

DON'T: Meet at venues where you're likely to be flooded with nostalgic 'wasn't it wonderful' memories and either fall into a weeping heap or a sizzling snog for the trade-off. Also, don't bother with anything that's not valuable or has no sentimental value – replace it with a newer, better one.

THE SITUATION: THE FIRST POST-BREAK-UP ENCOUNTER.

DO: Accept that you're probably going to hate how you look, even if you look fabulous. Let HIM say the first sentence after the initial greetings. Then casually say you'd love to talk (this is key – otherwise it looks like you are avoiding him), but you have to meet someone. Saunter off straight to the nearest phone to call your closest friend, telling her in detail what he was wearing, what he said, how he said it, etc.

DON'T: Start crying, laughing hysterically, talking non-stop or mauling him.

SITUATION: SEEING HIM TALKING (OR FLIRTING!) WITH ANOTHER WOMAN.

DO: Give him a teensy smile (as in, 'Uh-huh, got your number, dude'), nod and walk, don't run, straight to the nearest phone ... you know the drill.
DON'T: Approach him, find your own boy model to flirt with or collapse in a soppy, snivelling mess.

SITUATION: MEETING AT A PARTY AND, 'ACCIDENTALLY' GETTING TOGETHER.

DO: Accept that it happens. A lot. So don't dwell on it.
DON'T: Call him. What can you say to him that hasn't been said already? Think of it as your goodbye 'kiss'.

SITUATION: BUMPING INTO HIM AND HIS PRETTY NEW GIRLFRIEND.

DO: Smile. Be civil. Ask how he's doing. Say hi to the new babe. Then find that best friend. Unless, of course, you're with YOUR new guy. Who happens to look exactly like George Clooney (dream come true!). In which case, flaunt it.
DON'T: Be tempted to spill all the gory moments of your break-up to your new guy or his new girl. If either ask, just say, 'We used to go out.'

Nine Uses for an Ex-Boyfriend

Your relationship wasn't a total waste of time.

1 COMEBACK TO YOUR MOTHER: When she gives her 'Why aren't you married like all your sisters and cousins' speech, simply say, 'Well you didn't want me to marry that last loser, did you?'

2 WAKE-UP CALL: Keep a picture of your ex to remind yourself that you should be dating men who didn't skip a link in the evolutionary chain.

3 EXERCISE INCENTIVE: You'd rather detour miles than risk running into him on his old turf.

4 BLAME MAGNET: Make him the scapegoat for everything bad in your life – the backpack you can't find, the bad mood you're in, your addiction to KitKats.

5 URGE TO SPLURGE: Now you have the perfect excuse to toss out those old faded sheets.

6 STRESS RELIEF: Smash anything he left behind to smithereens.

7 ARTISTIC INSPIRATION: For your soon-to-be critically acclaimed work, entitled *Ex Out*.

8 WILD SEX

9 GETTING SMARTER: Relationship psychologists say the best thing an ex is good for is to figure out what traits you DON'T want in a boyfriend.

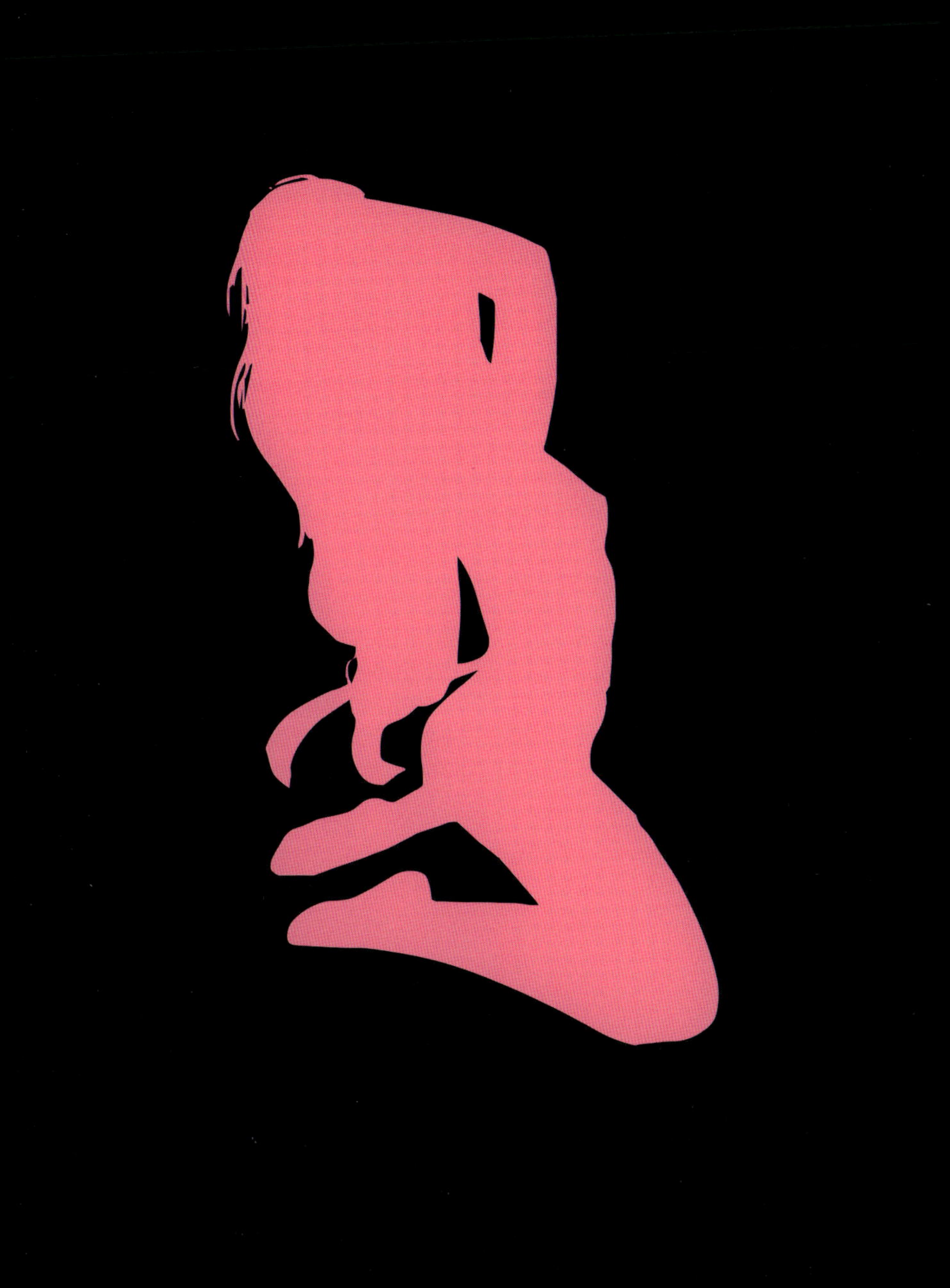

Acceptance

It happened and I'll live to love again.

OK, you're through to the final lap. You have acknowledged the plain fact that the relationship is over ('Whew, it's been six weeks since we ended it and I realized the other day I haven't thought about him for one whole day').

Most psychologists agree that during this process you learn to accept yourself and become ready to move on. You've vented your feelings, now it is time to go beyond merely surviving the heartbreak and figuring out how to avoid it in the future. This means:

1. Keeping a level head when it comes to dating

2. Taking an emotional inventory so you know what you want and expect out of your next relationship (quick fling versus real thing)

3. Most importantly, having faith – even if you are a vile wicked witch, there is an equally vile warlock out there for you.

Wrap It Up

You're finally over him when …

★ You genuinely hope he is happy when you hear he's with someone new.

★ You can go to what used to be your favourite restaurant, eat what used to be your favourite dish AND enjoy it.

★ He calls, saying he made a big mistake and wants you to come back, and you put him on hold to take a call from your mother.

★ You finally toss out all the love mementos – not because they cause you pain, but because you need the shelf space.

★ You compare New Guy to Ex-Guy and instead of thinking New Guy comes up short, you realize New Guy is a total upgrade from Ex-Guy ('Wow! Ex-Guy never gave me an hour-long back massage.' 'Huh! Ex-Guy never listened when I complained about work.' 'Mmm. Ex-Guy could never find my G-Spot.').

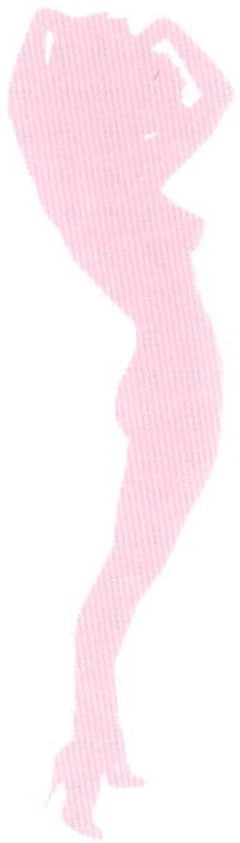

Singled Out

Why it's great to be single (honest).

★ You can flirt with your (incredibly cute) local bartender without your guy shooting green laser beams into your back.

★ You can spend the night drooling over Brad Pitt flicks without hearing a lot of snide remarks.

★ You can swap *Rush Hour 2*-meets-*American Pie* movies for chick flicks without guilt.

★ Did we mention flirting with your (incredibly cute) local bartender?

★ When you have sex with someone new, he doesn't wonder why you no longer want to do that kinky little thing he likes so much.

★ You get precious alone-time. In researching the effects of sensory deprivation, the ultimate solitude, Peter Suedfeld, PhD, a University of British Columbia psychologist who studies isolation, found that after just one hour of being totally on their own, people show lower blood pressure, higher mental functioning, enhanced creativity and a more positive outlook.

Lover Come Back

Do you really want him back? Take two or three weeks to think about restarting the connection. Suddenly being alone can feel terrible and alienating, and a lot of people have the knee-jerk reaction of wanting to make the loneliness go away by getting the other person back.

WHICH OF THE FOLLOWING THOUGHT PROCESSES BEST DESCRIBES YOUR CURRENT REALITY?

(a) It's not like I'm home every night sighing over him. It's been more than two weeks since we broke up. But I still dig him. And I can see where things went wrong and how we can work it out this time.
(b) Getting back together with my ex is better than being miserable and alone.
(c) I'm planning to dump his sorry ass the minute he takes me back.

It's (a) or nothing. Psychologists say if you have a life without your ex, but you've been thinking about your relationship and have realized that, uh, actually you still like him, you're thinking clearly. Ergo, your chances of staying together second time around are good. Any other answer means that you're still hurting. Get back together with him now, and you may never recover. And you'll probably kill a good deal of self-esteem as well.

If tip (a) holds true for you, then go for it. When Nancy Kalish, PhD, studied more than 500 couples that had called it quits, she found a surprising 72 per cent reunited and stayed together. The reason? They now had more realistic expectations of what they both wanted out of the relationship.

But wait at least a year. In the same study, Dr Kalish found that the longer a couple stayed apart, the more successful their reunion. Seems you need time to carve out your own identity and not be so-and-so's girlfriend for a while before you can truly decide if you WANT to be his arm jewellery again.

Love Turnaround

CAUTION: If he dumped you and is now creeping back, his reasons are not necessarily honourable.

★ He misses the sex. Hey, he's a man and he has needs! He wants his usual and customary style of loving with a partner he is familiar with. He feels safe with you and comfortable, because you know what he likes. But sex is not enough to keep a man – never has been and never will be. Things will deteriorate right back to square one because he is not there for the long haul, only a quick roll.

★ He needs to know you still care. In other words, he has seen you out on the town having a good time with some hot dude and needs to know he hasn't been replaced. His goal is to stay in contact with you and maintain your focus on him, just enough to keep the door open IN CASE he decides later that he wants to come back to you.

★ He doesn't want to start over. Thinking about the time he will need to spend trying to replace you is overwhelming. He thinks about the energy required to establish a foundation and framework for a new relationship and he gets a headache. He would rather apologize, give you what you want and just move on down the road with the woman who understands him and shares a history with him. Basically, he is lazy and would rather fight than switch.

★ He realizes he messed up bad. He has a chronic case of guilt. Now that he has had time away from you and the situation, he's come to the shocking realization that he truly cares for you (more than he knew). Don't keel over, it may be the dreaded 'L' word at work here! He has gone out, dated other women, hung out with his guy friends, and realized he isn't having the big fun he thought he would. He is depressed, unmotivated, moody and very unhappy. He comes to you to get back together when he is willing to make the adjustments and apologies and changes needed to return the relationship to its former level of focus and commitment, and move forward in love. To demonstrate his seriousness, he may make promises of a future and offer homes, cars, trips and wedding rings. In short, go for it.